YOU *CAN* BE WELL:

THE HOLISTIC NUTRITION GUIDE TO A HEALTHY, BALANCED LIFE

Ruth Thompson, RHN, MSW

Health E Guide
Cambridge, Ontario, Canada

A NOTE TO READERS

The information presented in this book is intended as a general reference for those who want to be proactive about their health and wellness. While the author offers recommendations to help prevent illness and address health issues of concern, no part of this book is intended to substitute for competent medical diagnosis, or as a prescription for the treatment of disease. For the diagnosis and treatment of any illness, you are advised to contact a licensed physician. It is especially important not to discontinue prescribed treatment or medication without the full concurrence of your doctor.

Copyright 2015 Ruth Thompson

Published by Health E Guide
Email: info@ruththompsonauthor.ca
Website: www.ruththompsonauthor.ca

Cover Design by Derek Thompson
Cover Photo by Nicole Peshnak

Canada Cataloguing in Publication Data
Thompson, Ruth, 1953-, author
You can be well: the holistic nutrition guide to a healthy, balanced life / Ruth Thompson.

Includes biographical references and index.
ISBN 978-0-9939588-0-9

1.   Nutrition 2. Holistic 3. Prevention 4. Wellness

Dedicated to the memory of my mother, Helene Brown Weaver,
who passed on her love of writing to me,
and
to my husband Derek and my children Jill and Travers,
for their love and support

Contents

ACKNOWLEDGEMENTS

This book is the result of years of study and practice in holistic health and nutrition, community development, and spiritual growth. Compiling and sharing what I have learned was always a goal. I had even started writing a couple of times but did not find the right formula. Then, in January 2012, my friend Heather Johnston asked me if we could meet each week to support each other's writing. It was these sessions with Heather that motivated me to keep going in the early stages, and helped me see this book through to its completion.

I wish to acknowledge the many researchers, authors, and practitioners in various fields whose groundbreaking work helped form the book's thesis, in particular Annemarie Colbin, Carolee Bateson-Cook, ND, Mary Enig, PhD, Sally Fallon, Raymond Francis, MSc, Ann Louise Gittleman, CNS, David Hawkins PhD, John Matsen, ND, and Michael Pollan.

I acknowledge with gratitude the permission to use quoted materials by Sally Fallon, Louise Hay, Carolyn Myss, PhD, Danielle Perrault, RHN, and Dr. Bernie Siegel.

I wish to thank my editor, Simone Gabbay, whose attention to detail and recommendations were critical to strengthening the message that I wished to convey.

Finally, I owe a great deal to my husband, Derek, for his support and patience during the three years it took me to write, refine, and edit this book. Writing is a solitary pursuit, but he kept me from being alone in it.

PREFACE

My passion for holistic nutrition emerged after my daughter, Jill, developed a mysterious, lingering ailment that defied diagnosis and treatment. Starting at age 12, she suffered through four years of low energy, nausea, and loss of mental ability; she functioned at about 60 percent capacity and lost her teen years to illness. Medical doctors were baffled because their tests found nothing to explain the illness. There were prescription drugs for symptom relief, but, with no tangible diagnosis, doctors eventually dismissed her condition as being "all in her head." I refused to accept this and looked at alternative health solutions. We consulted with holistic health practitioners, whose in-depth evaluations determined my daughter had a parasite, albeit one that was not considered a serious health threat. We were still left to wonder why she could not shake this benign intruder. It was later, through my studies in holistic nutrition, that I identified the most likely reasons for her lengthy parasitic infection. To that point in time, she had resisted eating vegetables and craved sugary treats; this would have compromised her overall health. On top of all that, just prior to exposure to the parasite, she had a vaccine that all children in Grade 7 received at that time. I considered it a strong possibility that this vaccine had challenged her immune system at precisely the wrong time.

Medical doctors' investigations had not considered her diet or the side effects from the vaccine. I became acutely aware of the limitations of a medical system that is overly reliant on tests and medications for symptom relief at the expense of thorough assessment of an individual's situation. Through my education and clinical experience in holistic nutrition, I now know that if my daughter's parasitic infection had been left untreated, her intestinal tract would have been damaged to the point of developing a serious bowel disease such as colitis or Crohn's disease, or indeed any chronic condition related to impaired immunity. Without holistic health solutions, I believe she would not be well today.

My daughter's ordeal is all too common. In my holistic nutrition consulting practice, I see numerous clients who have lingering ailments that cause undue suffering and interfere with their enjoyment of life. Frequently, as with my daughter, they have not made healthy nutritional choices. Before seeking my services, many relied on medications because they thought there were no other solutions. However, using holistic nutrition protocols, I could address their issues of concern, such as allergies, headaches, acid reflux, unexplained fatigue, and abdominal bloating.

In my clinical practice, I repeatedly witness dramatic health improvement after the appropriate changes in diet and lifestyle. My clients are surprised that such changes can do so much to restore their health. My message in this book is one of good news—you, too, can expect good health, to be well. There are simple changes that promote health now and prevent serious illness in the future.

I have poured all my knowledge and experience about holistic health into this book. I include the nutritional insights, assessment tools, and protocols that help my clients reach their health goals. If, at the time of my daughter's ordeal, I had known what I know now, her illness would not have dragged on for over four years. In my practice, I see children like her who, because their parents have embraced a holistic approach, can be well once again. I wish this for everyone.

A HOLISTIC MODEL OF WELLNESS

I believe many people settle for a state of health that is less than ideal. Minor health issues interfere with their enjoyment of life and, even though there is no diagnosable illness, they are not *well*. It is not enough *to be not sick*; we deserve to *be well*, which means living from day to day without undue concern, or medication needed, for a health or emotional issue. Another way to define *being well* is the physical and emotional state that allows us to fully engage in our lives—career, recreation, relationships. To *be well* is much more than physical health; it is about a mindset—making health-promoting choices *before* serious illness strikes, rather than afterward. *Being well* depends on doing everything possible to prevent illness in all its physical and emotional aspects. Unfortunately, few people experience what I am describing.

In North America, there is an alarming increase in the incidence of largely preventable health conditions such as asthma, digestive problems, overweight, and immune disorders. The statistics are alarming:

- In 2009, health statistics in the United States estimated that 24 million Americans suffered with asthma—almost triple the number compared to 1980.[1] The prevalence of asthma in Canada has risen dramatically over the last 20 years, now estimated by the Asthma Society of Canada to affect over three million Canadians.[2]

- Between 1995 and 2008, government statistics in both the United States[3] and Canada[4] showed a 70 percent increase in type 2 diabetes.

- Years after a declaration of "war on cancer" that triggered fundraising projects and research worldwide, the rate of cancer diagnoses has not decreased. Rather it is expected to increase.[5] The World Health Organization reports that cancer rates are highest in developed countries—the United States, Canada, Australia, France.[6]

- In 2004, cardiovascular disease was the leading cause of death in Canada, representing 32% of all deaths. The Public Health Agency of Canada reported "some progress in reducing the risk of developing CVD, and improving survival through effective management," but the agency also predicted a continued rise in cardiovascular disease because its major risk factor, obesity, is epidemic.[7]

All these health issues and illnesses are directly related to, and could be prevented by, diet and lifestyle choices. While there is more than enough evidence of these relationships, diet and lifestyle are not the focus of the North American health care system. Many authors and experts applaud prevention, but health systems afford it few resources. In 2003, the National Cancer Policy Board in the United States recommended increasing efforts to prevent cancer.[8] In a 2012 article in the

New England Journal of Medicine, two medical doctors labeled Western medicine as "sick care," and called for "re-engineering prevention into the U.S. system."[9] Despite this call for change, prevention receives little attention in medical practice in the United States and Canada; the focus continues to be on treating illnesses and relying on last-minute heroics to save people from dying.

In response to the current state of health care, I pose these critical questions:

Is it acceptable that people continue to suffer with asthma with no hope of a cure?

Is it okay to manage diabetes rather than seek to prevent it?

Is it enough to save people after a heart attack or a cancer diagnosis, while the rate of these life-threatening illnesses continues to climb?

Too many people have resigned themselves to being unwell because they believe there are no alternatives, when, in fact, there are. It is within our grasp to be well through a holistic health approach that focuses on broad determinants of health. The World Health Organization promotes a holistic approach in its definition of health "the complete physical, mental, and social well-being, and not merely the absence of disease or infirmity." This position is in line with what I propose—being well is much more than not being sick; it is about finding a healthy balance among the many influences on our health. The challenge is in knowing how to achieve this balance because of all the conflicting information, much of which comes from sources that seem reputable. The resulting confusion must be resolved—hence my motivation for writing this book.

Our quest to be well starts with an understanding of the roots of both health and ill health. What supports health? What challenges health? How can we naturally restore health after illness? Health is a function of multiple relationships among the body, mind, and spirit. In practical terms, good health requires more than a good diet; it is also about supportive social relationships, positive attitudes, a safe, toxin-free environment, and exercise. Equally important is how we respond to our diet and environment—our individual strengths and weaknesses. We may wonder why one person becomes ill, while another in the same situation does not. The answer lies in the differences in how our bodies function. For this reason, health status is not a simple equation of A + B = C. The creation of each person's health status is much more complex.

I propose a model of holistic health that explains how we can be well. My model is unique because it focuses on activities over which we have control. As something out of our control, genetic traits are not included in the model. In developing the Holistic Model of Wellness (Figure 1), I drew on my knowledge and experience in several fields: holistic nutrition, physiology, social policy, health care policy, psychology, community development, bioenergetics, and spirituality.

The Holistic Model of Wellness:

> Explains how health is a function of various influences;
>
> Explains individual differences in health outcomes;
>
> Promotes awareness of the roots of illness;
>
> Guides diet and lifestyle choices to prevent illness and help us be well;
>
> Provides a template for healing after health issues arise.

Within the model, there are three categories of influences on health:

> Choices—the health-related activities over which we have control;
>
> Responses—how the body responds to our choices;
>
> Outcomes—how we feel both physically and emotionally, i.e., energy.

Several inter-relationships exist among these influences, as depicted by the arrows in the model. The following is an introduction to choices, responses and outcomes, and their relationships to being well.

Figure 1: Holistic Model of Wellness

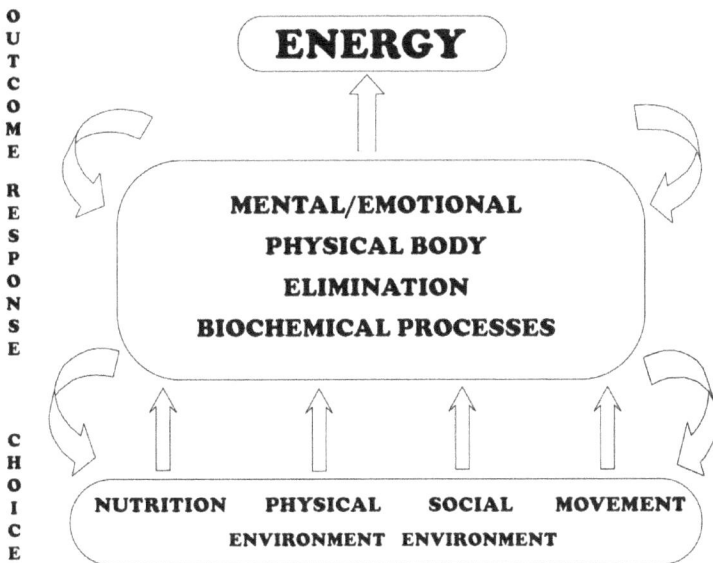

Choices

Every day we make choices about what we eat, where we live and work, with whom we associate, and how much we exercise. The relationship between unhealthy choices and disease are well known. In 2004, the Secretary of Health and Human Services in the United States made this statement: "…tobacco use, poor nutrition, and lack of physical activity are major contributors to the nation's leading killers.

America's poor eating habits and lack of physical activity are literally killing us."[10] In the model, I group health-related choices into four areas: *nutrition, physical environment, social environment,* and *movement.*

Nutrition relates to both the quantity and quality of our diet. Consuming poor-quality foods will negatively impact health, sooner or later. Unfortunately, in North America, even healthy foods (vegetables, fruits, and grains) have declined in quality. Agricultural methods and food processing give us nutrient-deficient foods and anti-nutrients that harm our health. The North American diet is rife with processed foods known to contribute to obesity and a host of illnesses. Another challenge is in the economic and political influences that dictate which foods are considered healthy. Myths about the health of some foods make nutritional choices even more difficult. Clarity on these issues will allow you to make dietary choices that are truly health-promoting.

Our **physical environment**—air, water, homes, workplaces, consumer products—contains synthetic chemicals, heavy metals, and infectious agents that can have serious health effects. Frequent travel and migration increases exposure to infectious agents such as bacteria, viruses, and parasites. Toxins are directly or indirectly related to chronic illness, such as cancer and autoimmune diseases. In this book, I identify the environmental threats of most concern in North America, their health effects, and how to avoid them.

Our **social environment** has a powerful effect on health, both emotionally and physically. The importance of supportive relationships is most clear when they are absent, such as in cases of abuse or neglect. Emotional scars from such experiences can increase the risk of physical illness and also be a barrier to healing. I draw on the extensive body of knowledge on how energy from emotional imbalances is involved in many common ailments—ulcers, high blood pressure, and irritable bowels.

Movement of the body keeps all its processes functioning optimally. Physical exercise lubricates joints, builds muscles, and strengthens bones, while lack of movement leads to atrophy of muscles and loss of bone mass. We see dramatic evidence of these effects in astronauts who spend several months on the International Space Station. Without exercise, bones weaken, are more easily broken, and we risk developing osteoporosis. Past injuries can limit movement and result in further deterioration in physical structure. I explore the complicated role of movement in health status, including too little and too much exercise.

Responses

There is no such thing as a truly "normal" individual—meaning average. We are all biochemically unique and need to be dealt with as such. ~ Jeffrey S. Bland, PhD[11]

Our choices about diet, environment, and movement are on one side of the equation. The other side is just as important—how our bodies respond. These body responses, essential to understanding our health status, can be grouped into four categories: *biochemical processes, elimination, physical body* and *mental/emotional.*

Biochemical processes include functions such as digesting food, absorbing nutrients, releasing neurotransmitters, activating immune cells, and maintaining hormone balance. Another word for these functions is metabolism, which refers to the processes within a living organism that maintain life. These processes are dynamic, never the same for long, and highly individual. Thanks to the work of scientist Roger J. Williams, we have known since the 1950s about "biochemical individuality"—foods on which we thrive may differ from those that are beneficial for someone else. Holistic nutrition holds the guiding principle that there is no one diet right for everyone. In this book, I offer the means to discovering the right diet for your needs.

You may have heard the expression *you are what you eat.* I maintain it is more accurate to say *you are what you eat and what you absorb.* Compromised nutrient absorption negates the benefits of a good diet and environment. Our ability to absorb nutrients, such as fats and minerals, can be impaired and result in nutrient deficiencies that increase the risk of illness. Faulty metabolism has been linked to serious health conditions such as heart disease, osteoporosis, and cancer. However, long before such illnesses develop, there will be warning signs in the form of bodily symptoms. It is critical to understand and act on such symptoms. My daughter suffered for four years with a parasite infection because health practitioners did not properly interpret and address her symptoms. Since then, I have dedicated my career to helping others avoid such suffering. In this book, I detail the bodily symptoms of most concern and, with this knowledge, how to take charge of your health.

Elimination is a critical response to our survival. We must eliminate waste—all the time. We expel carbon dioxide when breathing out, uric acid through the kidneys, solid waste through the bowels, and various toxins when we sweat. When we do not eliminate wastes well, they can be stored in the body and create toxic overload. Accumulation of toxins has been linked to diseases such as arthritis, cardiovascular disease, dementia, and cancer. In my nutrition practice, I observe that some of my clients are toxic because they are not efficient eliminators. While there is no medical test to detect poor elimination, symptoms alert us to this malfunction. I reveal the symptoms of poor elimination and toxic accumulation, as well as holistic nutrition protocols to address these issues.

The **physical body** responds to our choices of food, environment, and movement. The health of our physical body—bones, muscles, glands, and organs—is, in a real sense, a reflection of the quality of all our choices to date. Malfunction in other responses, such as digestion and elimination, can also lead to damage to body tissues and physical structure, which is visible in tests such as X-ray and CT scans. We have medical interventions to repair or replace some parts of the physical body (knees, hips, heart, etc.), but only after we suffer with ill health for a while. With a better understanding of dietary and lifestyle influences on the physical body, I believe we could avoid some restorative surgeries.

Mental/emotional responses have a powerful impact on our overall health; this is not new knowledge. Long ago, the Buddha said: "All that we are results from what we have thought. The mind is everything. What we think, we become." To every experience, we respond emotionally, either positively or negatively. Recent findings on the energy patterns of emotions explain how they can either benefit or harm our physical health. We have a choice about how we respond emotionally, but this hinges on being emotionally balanced. Based on my professional and personal experience, I offer principles for seeking balance in mental and emotional responses for being well.

Outcomes: Energy

Energy is the key indicator of life and the reflection of all our choices and body responses. When we have physical and emotional energy, we *are* well. Medical tests assess our health status using energy by means such as taking our body temperature, or by measuring activity in the nervous system (electroencephalogram or EEG) and the cardiovascular system (electrocardiogram or EKG). Magnetic resonance imaging (MRI) and the mammogram measure aberrant energy patterns that signal illness. But long before illness develops, the energy we feel both physically and emotionally is a reliable indicator of body function. Unexplained fatigue (not related to illness) is a symptom of body malfunction. In this book, I explain how holistic nutrition interventions can restore the energy needed to be well.

Dynamics of the Model

Our bodies are not just passive receivers of food and experiences. In the Holistic Model of Wellness, the arrows representing effects and responses go both ways—choices affect how our body responds and ultimately energy levels, but this can also work in reverse. Poor body responses can affect our choices. For example, with prolonged indigestion, the desire to eat can diminish and result in nutrient deficiencies and low energy. This happened to my daughter. She had recurrent nausea, became afraid to eat, which lead to nutrient deficiencies that delayed her healing. She also had no energy for exercise and lost muscle mass. If you suffer from an illness or depression, you may not feel up to preparing healthy meals or exercising. In this way, poor health begets poor health.

Need for a Holistic Model

The Holistic Model of Wellness explains what affects our health but also what we can do to maintain it. With this awareness, we do not have to wait until there is illness and disease to take action. This is a dramatic shift from the more common practice of making changes only after we become ill. In the long term, we cannot expect to *be well* if we rely on the "sick-care" model of health care, which has been the predominant approach by Western medicine over the past 100 years. If this approach were working, the quality of health in North America would be improving. Instead, the rate of diseases such as cancer, diabetes, and cardiovascular disease continue to rise. We can reverse these trends. The holistic approach that I propose will break the downward spiral into poor health. To underscore the importance of my message, there is the recent discovery of epigenetics. Rather than conceding that genetics control our health, epigenetics tells us that our choices can influence how our genes express in creating our health status. Unhealthy diet and lifestyle choices can effectively *turn on* genetic markers that increase risk of certain diseases. The good news!! Health-promoting choices can *turn off* these genes and prevent disease from developing.[12]

You will benefit from this book no matter your current health status. Perhaps you feel fairly well right now. You will learn how to continue to feel your best by understanding challenges to health and by following my holistic guidelines for the wellness of body, mind, and spirit. Perhaps you already suffer with some health issues—allergies, digestive problems, overweight, headaches—that appear to have no solution. For you, I provide holistic nutrition protocols that work to restore a healthy balance and prevent more serious illness. I divided this book into three parts, which I briefly outline.

Part 1: CHALLENGES TO BEING WELL

There are challenges to being well in North America related to the choices in the Holistic Model of Wellness—nutrition, physical environment, and social environment. To be well and prevent illness, it is critical to understand and act on these challenges. I devote four chapters to challenges in our food supply: farming methods and food handling (Chapter 1), the processing of food (Chapter 2), politics in nutrition research and food marketing (Chapter 3), and dispelling six prevailing food myths (Chapter 4). Chapter 5 details environmental toxins and how they can be involved in everything from minor health issues to serious illness. Chapter 6 discusses the powerful influence on physical health from social environment and emotional responses.

Part 2: HOLISTIC GUIDES TO BEING WELL

These three chapters form the central preventative information in this book. Chapter 7 outlines my holistic guide to quality food and how to avoid harmful toxins and infectious agents. Chapter 8 explains how to determine the right diet for your needs, and whether you have food sensitivities. Chapter 9 first gives a method for self-assessment of your emotional balance and then offers eight principles for balancing emotions I believe are foundations for being well.

Part 3: HOLISTIC GUIDES FOR RESTORING HEALTHY BALANCE

This part outlines the holistic nutrition approaches that I use to help my clients restore healthy balance after the onset of health conditions or illness. Understanding the natural healing process and how to support it is the first step (Chapter 10). In Chapter 11, I detail the holistic nutrition assessment tool of nutritional symptomatology, along with holistic nutrition interventions to deal with common digestive imbalances. Food is a powerful healing tool; in Chapter 12, I provide the healing diets and eating methods that aid in the recovery from almost any health concern. Chapter 13 presents the case for and against using nutritional supplements and when they support healing. In the final two chapters, I discuss the key therapeutic protocols in my holistic nutrition practice: cleansing (Chapter 14) and detoxification (Chapter 15).

This book offers a much-needed remedy to the current state of health in North America—rising rates of serious illness, chronic health conditions, and aging in sickness. We can make choices now that will reverse these trends. I conclude the book by summarizing my holistic health approach into ten guidelines that, if followed, will help you to *be well*.

Chapter Notes

1. United States, National Center for Health Statistics, "Asthma Prevalence, Health Care Use, and Mortality: United States 2005-2009" (January 2011): 32, accessed February 20, 2013, http://www.cdc.gov/nchs/data/nhsr/nhsr032.pdf.

2. "Asthma Facts and Statistics," *Asthma Society of Canada, asthma.ca,* accessed February 21, 2013, http://www.asthma.ca/corp/newsroom/pdf/asthmastats.pdf.

3. United States, Centers for Disease Control and Prevention, "Morbidity and Mortality Weekly Report: Increasing Prevalence of Diagnosed Diabetes — United States and Puerto Rico, 1995–2010," 61 no. 45 (November 16, 2012): 918-921, accessed March 1, 2013, http://www.cdc.gov/mmwr/preview/mmwrhtml/mm6145a4.htm.

4. Canada, Public Health Agency of Canada, "Diabetes in Canada: Facts and Figures from a Public Health Perspective," last modified December 15, 2011, http://www.phac-aspc.gc.ca/cd-mc/publications/diabetes-diabete/facts-figures-faits-chiffres-2011/highlights-saillants-eng.php#chp1.

5. "Worldwide Data," *World Cancer Research Fund International,* accessed November 13, 2014, http://www.wcrf.org/int/cancer-facts-figures/worldwide-data.

6. "GLOBOCAN 2012: Estimated Cancer Mortality and Prevalence in 2012," *World Health Organization, International Agency for Research on Cancer,* accessed May 4, 2014, http://globocan.iarc.fr/Pages/fact_sheets_cancer.aspx.

7. Canada, Public Health Agency of Canada, "2009 Tracking Heart Disease and Stroke in Canada" (June 10, 2009), accessed May 4, 2014, http://www.phac-aspc.gc.ca/publicat/2009/cvd-avc/report-rapport-eng.php.

8. National Cancer Policy Board, National Research Council of the National Academies, "Fulfilling the Potential of Cancer Prevention and Early Detection," Institute of

Medicine (April 2, 2003), accessed May 10, 2014,
http://www.iom.edu/reports/2003/fulfilling-the-potential-of-cancer-prevention-and-early-detection.aspx.

9. Farshad Fani Marvasti, MD and Randall S Stafford, MD, PhD. "From Sick Care to Health Care—Reengineering Prevention into the U.S. System," *New England Journal of Medicine*, 367 (September 6, 2012): 889-891, accessed May 12, 2014,
http://www.nejm.org/doi/full/10.1056/NEJMp1206230.

10. Tommy G. Thompson, Secretary, United States Department of Health and Human Services, "Testimony on Health and Wellness," *Presentation before the Senate Committee on Appropriations Subcommittee on Labor, Health and Human Services, Education* (July 15, 2004), accessed September 6, 2014, http://www.hhs.gov/asl/testify/t040715a.html.

11. Jeffrey S. Bland, "Introduction to 1998 Edition," ix, in *Biochemical Individuality: The Basis of the Genotrophic Concept,* by Roger J. Williams (New Canaan, Connecticut: Keats Publishing).

12. Sang-Woon Choi and Simonetta Friso, "Epigenetics: A New Bridge between Nutrition and Health," *Advances in Nutrition* 1 (November 2010): 8-16, accessed September 7, 2014, http://advances.nutrition.org/content/1/1/8.full.

PART 1: CHALLENGES TO BEING WELL

In Part 1, my aim is to convey how important your choices are in determining how well you can be. There are widespread challenges to being well in North America. Understanding these challenges is the first step to making health-supportive choices as outlined in the Holistic Model of Wellness—nutrition, physical environment, movement, and social environment. The effects of movement on health are addressed in Part 2 and Part 3.

1: FOOD PRODUCTION PERILS

Overall, vitamin and mineral content of American fruits and vegetables have declined significantly during the last fifty years. ~ Paul Bergner

Even if we eat the "right" foods, there is no assurance that these foods are nutritious. In this chapter, I reveal the extent of nutritional deficits in our food because of the prevailing food production practices. Our food goes on an unbelievable journey from the farm to our table that negatively affects food's nutritional value. Not only do modern farming methods reduce nutrients in food crops, they expose us to chemicals that pose health risks. Crop staples have also been modified, resulting in foods that our bodies may not recognize. The nutrient value of food can be reduced during transportation, storage, and cooking. Understanding all these challenges is the first step in ensuring our diet is truly health supportive.

Health Risks from 21st-Century Farming

Farming methods have changed radically in the past century. Innovators in crop science perhaps made changes with the best of intentions to increase crop yields to feed a burgeoning population. However, some new methods have not resulted in improved food quality.

Animal husbandry in North America has become about mass production to serve consumer demand and make a profit, and less about high-quality meat and poultry. Large-scale operations speed up maturation of the animals, so they get to the slaughterhouse faster. Growth hormones may be used that compromise the health of the livestock and the health of those consuming the resulting meat products. Large-scale operations fatten cattle in huge feedlots and house chickens in cramped quarters. These conditions are not healthy for the animals, and many get sick. As a result, these operations must use antibiotics to prevent death of livestock before they are due for slaughter. Overuse of antibiotics in our food animals has been linked to the rise of antibiotic-resistant strains of bacteria, so-called "super bugs." I highly recommend the documentary film *Food, Inc.* for the inside scoop on industrialized farming methods and their effects on the quality of meat and poultry.[1]

Modern crop agriculture is based on chemicals: fertilizers, pesticides, herbicides, and fungicides. Our ancestors did not have these chemicals. They used manure for fertilizer and fought off diseases and pests the best way they could. However, insects and plant diseases damaged their crops; weeds stunted plant growth. Farmers were naturally eager to reduce their economic losses from weeds and pests and readily embraced chemical agriculture. On the surface, these modern farming methods seem like progress, but there have been significant nutritional costs to the consumer.

Chemical fertilizers help crops grow fast and may even make them look healthy. However, fertilized crops will lack vital nutrients. The book *Real Food for a Change* explains how this happens. "The chemical fix institutes growth so fast and furious that it sacrifices the slow and steady uptake of complex nutrients…the growth spurt fuelled by synthetic fertilizers leaves calcium, magnesium and zinc—all crucial to heart, bone and mental health—in the dust."[2] In their 1990 book *Empty Harvest,* Mark Anderson and the late Dr. Bernard Jensen alerted us to the alarming effects of chemical fertilizers—vegetables and fruits with little nutritional value and elevated sodium content. This is not new information—studies over the past 60 years have consistently shown that any crop that is chemically fertilized is more apt to be nutritionally deficient.[3] In short, we may have wonderfully large and brightly coloured produce, but it contains a fraction of the nutrients that it should, and sodium at levels that increase our risk of cardiovascular disease.

Pesticides approved for use on crops years ago are now proving to have severe health effects:

- The United States Environmental Protection Agency (EPA) has been evaluating the health risks of pesticides since 1986 and has programs in place to warn of health risks from overexposure.[4]
- In a 2004 review of research on the health risks from pesticide exposure, the Ontario College of Family Physicians reported links to cancer, neurological and reproductive problems, and recommended that people limit their exposure to pesticides.[5]
- A study in 2006 found that Canadian women who had worked in farming in their lives were three times more likely to develop breast cancer than women who had not been involved in farming.[6]
- The National Pesticide Information Center (United States) states that "…pesticides by their nature are toxic to some degree. Even the least-toxic products, and those that are natural or organic, can cause health problems if someone is exposed to enough of it."[7]

Defenders of pesticides claim that residue on crops is too low to cause health problems. However, there is evidence that we are absorbing pesticides, and that health issues may result. A study in 2003 found that children who ate conventionally grown produce had pesticide residue in their bodies six times higher than children who ate 70 percent organic food.[8] Another study in 2010 found that children with attention deficit hyperactivity disorder (ADHD) had higher levels of pesticide residue in their bodies than children without ADHD.[9] This association does not prove that pesticides cause ADHD, but given the widespread agreement on the ill effects from pesticides, there should be cause for alarm. Consider this: If children already have residue in their bodies, imagine what older individuals have accumulated, and the health problems they could suffer.

The Case for Organic

If you think washing conventional produce will do it, think again. Environmental Working Group analyzed pesticide residue on fruits and vegetables in Canada only to find that many soft-skinned fruits and vegetables absorb these toxins into their flesh. This means we cannot wash off toxins. EWG found some produce more prone to pesticide residue than others, as follows:

Highest in pesticide residue:

Fruits: peaches, apples, strawberries, nectarines, pears, cherries, red raspberries

Vegetables: spinach, bell peppers, celery, potatoes, hot peppers

Lowest in pesticide residue:

Fruits: avocados, bananas, papaya, pineapples, kiwi, mangos

Vegetables: asparagus, broccoli, cauliflower, corn, onions, peas[10]

The best way to avoid pesticide residue is to eat organic produce. In Canada and the United States, there are organic standards to limit the use of pesticides on crops, but standards are not as strict in some Central and South American countries. Another good reason to eat organic produce is its nutritional value. A review of over 300 studies of the nutrient content of organic crops revealed significantly higher levels of antioxidants known to be critical to health. Of the five antioxidants studied, organic crops had between 19 to 51 percent higher levels compared to non-organic crops.[11]

Modified Foods

There is a long tradition of modifying food crops, and with few concerns about health effects. The 19th-century monk Gregor Mendel discovered plants passed their genetic traits to the next generation. This led to selective breeding, or hybridizing, of plants with more desirable characteristics. Hybridizing plants has continued to this day to suit human tastes—a juicier tomato, a larger potato, etc.

Wheat is one crop that modern-day crop scientists have hybridized, but not without ill effects on human health. The intention was to produce hardier variety with a shorter growing time and flour that makes lighter bread. In the process of implementing these changes, the gluten content of wheat has increased sharply. Today's version of the popular grain is not the same food that people ate 30 years ago. Since these changes, there has been a dramatic increase in gluten intolerance and sensitivities to wheat. According to cardiologist Dr. William Davis, author of the book *Wheat Belly: Lose the Wheat, Lose the Weight, and Find Your Path Back to Health,* modern wheat is causing many health problems, including overweight, weight around the middle, colitis, insulin resistance, diabetes, high blood pressure, high cholesterol, accelerated aging, skin rashes, and disorders of the nervous system. Dr. Davis refers to wheat as "head-to-toe destruction of health."[12] Chapters 2 and 4 further discuss what we have done to wheat, its health effects and its role in a quality diet.

Genetically Modified Food

Hybridization involves mating of plants from the same family, but genetic modification (GM) is a newer and completely different process; genes from one species are inserted into another—a process that would never occur in nature. Work on GM foods began in the 1980s. A pioneer in the field, Scotland-based scientist Arpad Pusztai, found that rats eating GM potatoes had immune system problems and underdeveloped organs. In his book, *Secret Ingredients: The Brave New World of Industrial Farming,* Stuart Laidlaw reports on Pusztai's research and the resulting bad publicity that led to the European consumers' refusal to eat GM foods.[13] Unfortunately, the European experience has not deterred the development of GM crops in North America.

Laidlaw refers to two classes of genetically modified crops:

"Herbicide resistant plants, such as soybeans, canola or corn that can be sprayed with powerful weed killers and not die, e.g., 'Roundup Ready Corn'"

"Insect-resistant plants, such as corn or cotton, that contain the *Bt* gene, which means they can produce their own toxin" [14]

Glyphosate is the chemical name for the herbicide, brand name Roundup®, which is now in widespread use in North America in the crops that Laidlaw mentions. Wheat is another crop that farmers may spray with this herbicide prior to harvest. Crops can be sprayed liberally with the herbicide—weeds die but the crop survives.

To make crops naturally toxic to insects, researchers in North America started inserting the *Bacillus thuringiensis*, or *Bt* gene, into crops. *Bt* is a naturally occurring bacterial disease of insects that would not naturally be present in plants. The addition of the *Bt* gene to corn means that it produces its own insecticide; no spraying is required. *Bt* corn looks beautiful and is worm-free, making it very attractive to consumers. Almost all corn reaching our tables in North America is the genetically modified *Bt* variety. If you think avoiding corn is the answer, be aware that many processed foods use corn derivatives as sweeteners. Food manufacturers in North America use corn sweeteners extensively because they are much cheaper than sugar cane, which must be imported.

From the beginning, proponents of GM food claimed that GM is very precise and predictable. However, the findings in the Human Genome Project in 2001 does not support this claim. The project researchers were surprised to find that human genes act in combinations to produce character traits. There is no one gene to control eye or hair colour, for instance. This shows that genes work in combination in all living things.[15] What does this mean for genetic modification? It will be impossible to predict how changing one gene in a food affects its nutrient profile. For all we know, the result is a foreign substance that our bodies do not recognize as food. We may not know the long-term effects on health from eating GM foods for several years. Just as it took years to prove the adverse health effects of smoking tobacco, we may not understand the effects of GM foods until many people have suffered ill effects.

Research evidence of harm to human health from GM foods has not been compelling enough to ban their use in North America. However, the EPA has set acceptable limits for exposure to glyphosates. They state that long-term exposure over such limits can cause kidney damage and reproductive problems.[16] A recent journal article by researchers Anthony Samsel and Stephanie Seneff propose that, based on known effects of glyphosate on certain enzymes and proteins, exposure to the herbicide may be the "most important causal factor" in rising rates of celiac disease and gluten intolerance.[17] Research has yet to confirm their theory. A study in 1999 found adverse health effects of Bt corn pollen on butterflies.[18] It is likely this finding was downplayed because *Bt* corn represented only 19 percent of the corn crop in the United States at the time.[19] However, by 2009, *Bt* corn represented 63 percent of corn in production.[20] This raises the question whether we can expect increased health risks to butterflies and humans. To date, there is not enough solid evidence against GM foods. A review of several studies concluded: "Most studies with GM foods indicate that they may cause hepatic, pancreatic, renal, and reproductive effects and may alter hematological [blood], biochemical, and immunologic parameters, the significance of which remains to be solved with chronic toxicity studies."[21]

There is a grass-roots movement against GM foods in the United States and Canada. The Non-GMO Project raises awareness of the health risks of GM foods and lobbies for labelling of foods containing GMOs. This non-profit organization warns the *Bt* toxin in GM insecticidal crops may be toxic or an allergen, and cautions us on the impact of toxic residue from the herbicide Roundup. On their website, they report that the most common GM foods are soy, cotton, canola, corn, sugar beets, Hawaiian papaya, alfalfa, and squash (zucchini and yellow).[22] This list includes both types of GM foods: insect-resistant and herbicide-resistant crops.

Despite a growing body of evidence and organized opposition to GM foods, industry and government support continues. Health Canada continues to approve *Bt* corn as safe for human consumption. Until there is some regulation or labelling, the best way to avoid GM foods is to eat organic produce.

Food Transportation

My grandparents were farmers who grew almost all their own vegetables and fruits and preserved them for the winter. Two generations later, most of my family are city dwellers with year-round access to imported produce from anywhere in the world. In Canada, we rely on imported food for eight or nine months of the year. Unfortunately, long-distance transportation of food reduces its nutrient content. To avoid being overripe, farmers pick fruits while still green, which means the fruits may never reach their full nutrient content.

Once produce is harvested, its nutrient level immediately declines. Long transit rides are almost a guarantee of nutrient-deficient food. When we buy produce, it may be a nice bright colour (green, red, orange), but after several days in transit, it is not likely to be very nutritious. During transit, food is at risk of infestation from insects, pests, bacteria, fungi, and viruses. To prevent such infestation, food is irradiated. Radioactive materials create an energy field that kills bugs and bacteria. Critics claim that this changes the chemical composition of the food and negatively affects human health. While irradiation promises to save a great deal of money for the farmer, retailer, and even the consumer, the verdict is not in about potential health effects from the practice.

Food Storage

Since the invention of refrigerators and freezers, we have stored food much longer than in the past. Every day we store fresh food means nutrient losses. In some parts of the world, daily shopping trips for fresh produce are a common practice. This is the best way to ensure optimal nutrition, but only if the produce is not transported long distances. Produce frozen at its peak of freshness is more apt to have the desired nutrition than fresh produce that sits in a truck for several days. During the growing season, local produce is the best choice.

Food containers can also affect the health of food and fluids. In my mother's memoirs from the 1930s, she described how they stored food in either glass jars or wooden bins. Today almost everything comes to us in plastic, boxes or cans. Food that is in contact with these containers can be adversely affected. Plastics, which are derived from petroleum, are hardly benign packaging. Some plastic residues can get into food or fluids. It is well known in the holistic health field that compounds in plastics are a source of *xenoestrogens* (*xeno* meaning fake) which can disrupt female hormones. Environmental Working Group warns of the ill effects on male hormones from chemicals found in plastics called *phthalates*.[23]

Concerns about the effects of plastics in food containers have recently been validated. In 2008, researchers discovered that *Bisphenol A* (BPA) in plastic bottles and the lining of cans was a potential hazard to health. BPA could leak out of the can linings into food and migrate from polycarbonate plastic bottles into food or fluids. To date, the primary concern has been the health risks to young children. Health Canada's position on BPA in 2008 was one of cautious concern. They stated:

"Current dietary exposure to BPA through food packaging uses is not expected to pose a health risk to the general population, including newborns and infants. However, due to the uncertainty raised in some animal studies relating to the potential effects of low levels of BPA, the Government of Canada is taking action to enhance the protection of infants and young children."[24]

More recently, WebMD reports:

"The FDA [Food and Drug Administration] maintains that studies using standardized toxicity tests have shown BPA to be safe at the current low levels of human exposure. But based on other evidence—largely from animal studies—the FDA expressed "some concern" about the potential effects of BPA on the brain, behavior, and prostate glands in fetuses, infants, and young children."[25]

During 2013 and 2014, the FDA banned BPA from baby bottles, *Sippy* cups and infant formula packaging.[26]

Many manufacturers have voluntarily eliminated BPA from plastic containers, but the fact remains that we were already exposed for several years. The long-term effects remain unclear. The alternatives to plastic food containers are cans, stainless steel, or glass. Cans expose us to tin solder and aluminum; both have adverse health effects, which are discussed in Chapter 5. However, most cans (approximately 80 percent) are lined with plastic. While plastics containing BPA are gone, I post this question: *Is there another toxic threat from plastics yet to be identified?*

Cooking

Cooking is the last nutritional cost exacted on our food. Deep-frying is perhaps the greatest insult because it produces artery-clogging fats. Barbecued meat that is charred produces cancer-causing carcinogens. Boiling vegetables leaches their nutrients into the cooking water. Cooking in aluminum pans can expose us to this toxic heavy metal. To ensure maximum nutrient content, many nutritionists recommend minimal cooking and some promote eating only raw fruits and vegetables. However, a completely raw diet is not practical for everyone, and can aggravate digestive problems, such as irritable bowel syndrome. In addition, the properties of food can change during cooking. Cruciferous vegetables (broccoli, cauliflower, Brussels sprouts) contain goitrogens in raw form that cooking breaks down. Goitrogens can depress thyroid function—of particular concern for those with low thyroid, i.e., hypothyroid. For these reasons, a balance of raw and cooked vegetables is appropriate for most people. Ideal cooking methods are presented in Chapter 7: Quality Food and Toxin-Free Living. In Chapter 12: Use Food for Healing, I further discuss the issues related to raw foods.

In summary, you can avoid food production perils by eating food that is
-as close to nature as possible;
-organically grown;
-not genetically modified;
-not transported long distances, which causes nutrient losses;
-prepared in ways that retain nutrients (vitamins, mineral, and enzymes).
Unfortunately, there are other threats to food quality due to refining and additives. These are addressed in the next chapter.

Chapter Notes

1 . *Food, Inc.,* DVD, Directed by Robert Kenner (Magnolia Pictures, 2008).

2. Wayne Roberts, Rod MacRae and Lori Stahlbrand, *Real Food for a Change: Bringing Nature, Joy and Justice to the Table* (Toronto, Ontario: Random House, 1999), 19.

3. Dr. Bernard Jensen and Mark Anderson, *Empty Harvest: Understanding the Link between Our Food, Our Immunity, and Our Planet* (New York, New York: Penguin Putnam, 1990), 77-8.

4. United States, Environmental Protection Agency, "Assessing Pesticide Cumulative Risk," last modified June 2, 2014, http://www.epa.gov/pesticides/cumulative/.

5. Margaret Sanborn, MD et al., "Systematic Review of Pesticide Human Health Effects," *The Ontario College of Family Physicians* (2004), accessed June 6, 2014, http://ocfp.on.ca/docs/public-policy-documents/pesticides-literature-review.pdf.

6. James T. Brophy et al., "Occupation and Breast Cancer: A Canadian Case–Control Study," *Annals of New York Academy of Sciences* 1076 (2006): 765–77, accessed September 6, 2014, http://www.ncbi.nlm.nih.gov/pubmed/17119253.

7. Oregon State University and United States Environmental Protection Agency, "Pesticides and Human Health," *National Pesticide Information Center,* last modified March 11, 2014, http://npic.orst.edu/health/humhealth.html.

8. Cynthia Curl et al., "Organophosphorus pesticide exposure of urban and suburban preschool children with organic and conventional diets," *Environmental Health Perspectives* 111 no.3 (March 2003): 377–82 accessed March 25, 2014, http://www.ncbi.nlm.nih.gov/pmc/articles/PMC1241395/.

9. Maryse F. Bouchard et al., "Attention-Deficit/Hyperactivity Disorder and Urinary Metabolites of Organophosphate Pesticides," *Pediatrics Online (*May 17, 2010), accessed March 20, 2014, doi: 10.1542/peds.2009-3058.

10. "EWG's 2014 Shoppers Guide to Pesticides in Produce," *Environmental Working Group,* (April 2014), accessed September 10, 2014, http://www.ewg.org/foodnews/.

11. Marcin Baranski, et al., "Higher antioxidant and lower cadmium concentrations and lower incidence of pesticide residues in organically grown crops: a systematic literature review and meta-analyses," *British Journal of Nutrition* 112 no.5 (September 2014): 794-811, accessed September 10, 2014, http://www.ncbi.nlm.nih.gov/pubmed/24968103.

12. William Davis, MD, *Wheat Belly: Lose the Wheat, Lose the Weight, and Find Your Path Back to Health* (New York, New York: Rodale Books, 2011), 41.

13. Stuart Laidlaw, *Secret Ingredients: The Brave New World of Industrial Farming* (Toronto: McClelland & Stewart Ltd., 2003), 92-5.

14. Ibid., 97.

15. Laidlaw, *Secret Ingredients*, 102-3.

16. United States, Environmental Protection Agency, "Technical Fact Sheet on: Glyphosates," accessed December 9, 2014, http://www.epa.gov/ogwdw/pdfs/factsheets/soc/tech/glyphosa.pdf.

17. Anthony Samsel and Stephanie Seneff, "Glyphosate, Pathways to Modern Diseases II: Celiac Sprue and Gluten Intolerance," *Interdisciplinary Toxicology* 6 no.4 (March 2014): 159-184, accessed December 9, 2014, DOI: 10.2478/intox-2013-0026.

18. John E. Losey, et al., "Transgenic pollen harms monarch larvae," *Nature* 399, no.6733 (May 20, 1999): 214-5, accessed April 20, 2014, doi:10.1038/20338.

19. Tom Clarke, "Monarchs Safe from *Bt*," *Nature* 10, no.1038 (September 12, 2001), accessed April 20, 2014, www.nature.com/news/2001/010912/full/news010913-12.html.

20. Jan Suszkiw, United States Department of Agriculture, "New Study Shows *Bt* Corn of Benefit to Farmers," *U.S. News & World Report* (October 12, 2010) accessed October 15, 2014, http://www.usnews.com/science/articles/2010/10/12/new-study-shows-benefits-of-bt-corn-to-farmers.

21. A. Dona, and I.S. Arvanitoyannis, "Health risks of genetically modified foods," *Critical Reviews in Food Science and Nutrition,* 49 (2009): 164–75, accessed March 2, 2014, http://www.ncbi.nlm.nih.gov/pubmed/18989835.

22. "GMOs and Your Family," *Non-GMO Project, Nongmoproject.org,* accessed March 5, 2014, http://www.nongmoproject.org/.

23. "Dirty Dozen Endocrine Disruptors," *Environmental Working Group* (October 28, 2013) http://www.ewg.org/research/dirty-dozen-list-endocrine-disruptors

24. Canada, Health Canada, "Food and Nutrition: Bisphenol A" (December, 2010) accessed March 2, 2014, www.hc-sc.gc.ca/fn-an/securit/packag-emball/bpa/index-eng.php.

25. "health-e-head2toe: How Environmental Exposure May Affect Your Child," *WebMD,* accessed December 5, 2014, http://www.webmd.com/children/environmental-exposure-head2toe/bpa.

26. United States, Food and Drug Administration, "Bisphenol A (BPA): Use in Food Contact Application" (November 2104), accessed December 5, 2014, http://www.fda.gov/NewsEvents/PublicHealthFocus/ucm064437.htm.

2: WHAT ELSE CAME TO DINNER

Most people view malnutrition as an issue exclusive to third-world countries, where there is not enough food to eat but malnutrition exists in North America and it is primarily because of food processing. A dentist, the late Dr. Weston A. Price, first opened our eyes to the negative impact of the modern diet on our health. From his work in the 1920s and 30s, Dr. Price found that people who had embraced the "modern" diet of processed foods had markedly more tooth decay than those who stayed with a traditional diet. In *Diet and Nutrition: A Holistic Approach*, Dr. Rudolph Ballantyne highlights a more important aspect of Dr. Price's discovery: poor diet results in a "decay of health," including deformed facial bones, lower IQs, personality disorders, higher incidence of degenerative diseases, and birth defects.[1] Dr. Price suspected something was missing in the modern diet that caused these health problems. Today we know that the modern diet is deficient in several nutrients due, in part, to our farming methods (see Chapter 1), but also because of food processing and additives—preservatives, artificial flavours, and colours.

In North America, there is a ready supply of highly processed convenience foods containing refined grains, sugar, additives, and damaged fats. This way of eating, commonly referred to as the Standard American Diet (SAD), is recognized as contributing to the *epidemics* of obesity, cardiovascular disease, diabetes, cancer, and osteoporosis.[2] In the 1970s, the Select Committee on Nutrition and Human Needs in the United States reported on deficiencies of the modern diet and threats to human health. Chair of the Committee, Senator George McGovern, made the stunning statement that "six of the ten leading causes of death in the United States have been linked to our diet."[3] Unfortunately, these warnings from 40 years ago have not led to dramatic improvements in food quality or reduced popularity of the SAD. The specific challenges arising from this diet are addressed in this chapter.

Convenience Eating

In the late sixties, my parents went away for the weekend, leaving TV dinners for my teenage brother and me. No one, including my parents, knew the health dangers from these highly processed "meals"—refined flour, unhealthy fats, artificial flavours, and preservatives. Since then, convenience foods have become commonplace in the North American diet to the detriment of our health.

Because of our desire for convenience, we are participants in the decline in food's value. People work long hours and with more dual-income families, there is little time to prepare home-cooked meals. In response, food companies have developed easy-to-prepare meals: microwavable dinners, frozen entrees, and boxed meals—all highly processed and nutritionally deficient. Fast food is another popular dinner option for families—another source of processed food. Statistics Canada reports that drive-through, takeout, and delivery services in Canada have increased from 53 percent of all food-service meals in 1994 to 61 percent in 2004. The most popular fast food is likely the least healthy food: French fries.[4]

Unfortunately, fast food is missing vital nutrients. The 2004 documentary film, *Super Size Me,* graphically depicts the effects of nutrient-deficient fast foods. In the film, the protagonist voluntarily eats only fast food for 30 days. He exacts this bizarre experiment on himself to see what would happen to his health. Early in the experiment, he feels fatigued and sick all the time. At 21 days, the doctor advises him to stop the experiment because of potential damage to his liver. By the end of his 30-day experiment, he also gained 30 pounds.[5] Since this film's release, the fast-food restaurant in question stopped its "super-size" option and started offering healthier menu items. It is likely the negative publicity from the film was the catalyst for these changes. As consumers, we have some power. The threat of lost business is a great incentive for food companies to improve the quality of their products.

Refined Foods

Wheat and sugar are two foods whose nutritional value is reduced by refining. When wheat is refined to produce "white flour," the bran and the germ are removed. The bran is the source of fibre in wheat. The germ contains most of the nutritional benefits of wheat, such as protein, B vitamins and omega-3 fatty acids. Without fatty acids, which are very prone to spoilage, refined wheat stays fresh much longer than whole wheat. Fatty acids are available from other food sources and are therefore not the concern. It is the lack of B vitamins in refined, white flour that produce serious health effects.

In the early days of refined wheat consumption, epidemics of beriberi and pellagra resulted. These illnesses are because of severe deficiencies of vitamins B1 and B3 respectively, both of which are lost during refining process to make white flour. It was not until the 1930s that scientists identified what was missing and millers started adding B vitamins to refined wheat. By the 1990s, public health authorities realized that bread also needed to be fortified with folic acid. The addition of B vitamins is not a perfect replacement for what was lost during refining. Consumers of refined wheat are at risk of B vitamin deficiencies, which affect several body systems: nervous (e.g., insomnia, anxiety, depression, memory loss), digestive (indigestion, constipation, and low blood sugar), circulatory (high cholesterol) and reproductive (menstrual issues). Folic acid is well known for its importance in fetal brain development.[6]

Today, commercial bakeries are producing whole-wheat breads. However, most whole-wheat products still contain some refined flour. I learned this firsthand from someone who works in the wheat wholesale industry in Canada. The label may say "whole-wheat" but this seems to mean that whole-wheat is present not that it is the only grain source. The only way to be sure that a product is exclusively whole grain is to look for "100% whole grain" on the label.

Sugar is the other refined food with negative health effects. Refined sugar is an *empty-calorie* food, which means it contains calories, but no nutrients. Sugar cane, the source of refined, white sugar, contains B vitamins and several minerals, including calcium and potassium. These are all lost during the refining process. When we eat empty calorie foods such as refined sugar, our bodies, being highly tuned to nutrient levels, will signal us to eat more food to provide needed nutrients. This is how eating excess sugar is linked to overeating and ultimately overweight. Besides making us gain weight, too much sugar carries several health risks. There are numerous studies about the ill effects of eating too much sugar. In the 2014 book *Fat Chance: Beating the Odds against Sugar, Processed Foods, Obesity and Disease*, Dr. Robert H. Lustig, with extensive research backing his every word, gives us the "bitter truth" about sugar: it is the driving force behind obesity and a cluster of chronic metabolic diseases, such as type-2 diabetes, hypertension, high cholesterol, heart disease, and kidney disease.[7] Cancer, too, is a disease that feeds off sugar.

The amount of sugar we consume is a concern to many health experts and nutritionists. Over the past century, North Americans have overloaded their diets with sugar, mostly because of the sugar content of processed foods. Food activist Michael Pollan reports that, since 1909, the percentage of calories from sugars in the American diet increased from 13 percent to 20 percent.[8] Dr. Lustig identifies the last half of the twentieth century as the period when sugar intake increased to the point of affecting human health. He points the finger specifically at high-fructose corn syrup.[9]

A popular sugar source in North America because corn is readily available and inexpensive, high-fructose corn syrup may have worse health effects than refined white sugar derived from sugar cane. In 2010, a Princeton University research team showed sweeteners are not equal when it comes to weight gain. Rats fed high-fructose corn syrup gained significantly more weight than those eating table (i.e., white) sugar. Long-term consumption of high-fructose corn syrup also led to a rise in circulating blood fats called triglycerides. The researchers believe their work explains the dramatic rise in obesity in the United States.[10] Consumption of high-fructose corn syrup has been implicated in several health conditions:[11]

Accelerated aging

Insulin resistance

Type 2 diabetes

Diabetic complications (loss of eyesight, kidney disease, circulation problems)

Non-alcoholic fatty liver disease

Hyperuricemia—related to the development of gout

Abnormally high triglyceride levels—implicated in cardiovascular disease

Diets high in sugar will depress the immune system. As mentioned in the preface of this book, my daughter had a parasitic infection that became chronic, and I deemed this was in part, because she gravitated to sugary foods. My son recovered quickly from his exposure to the same parasite. One difference between them was diet—my daughter had too much sugar in her diet, while my son did not. It became clear that my daughter's nutritional foundation was so poor that it had weakened her immunity to the point she was more susceptible to the parasite than her brother was. This caught up to her by age 12. I ask you to consider the negative health effects of such eating patterns over longer periods.

Food Additives

Processed food contains additives that preserve, sweeten, or colour our food. Naturopath and health advocate, Janet Starr-Hull, estimates that there are 14,000 synthetic chemicals in our food supply and few have been tested for their safety.[12] Of particular concern is the role of chemical food additives, such as artificial sweeteners and colouring agents, in the emergence of attention deficit hyperactivity disorder (ADHD). One study funded by the European Union Food Safety Authority found that a combination of several additives triggered ADHD symptoms in children.[13] The European Union leads the way in regulating the food industry to reformulate children's food products. In North America, there is less regulatory concern about additives—it is up to consumers to become educated label readers. Three types of additives have potential negative health effects: artificial dyes, artificial flavours, and preservatives.

Artificial Dyes

Red, blue, and yellow dyes are all added to food in North America. Of most concern is *tartrazine*, also known as Yellow Dye #5, which is related to allergic reactions and asthma attacks. Austria, Finland, Sweden, and Norway have banned *tartrazine*, but in North America, it colours many food products, such as macaroni-and-cheese dinners, chewing gum, gelatin desserts, popsicles, and ice cream. It may also be present in foods we consider healthy, such as cheese, fruit juices, and cow's milk. Over-the-counter drugs may also contain *tartrazine* as a colouring agent. Red and blue dyes can also cause health problems.

My assessments using the Bioenergetic Evaluation (see Appendix 1) with many clients revealed numerous instances of sensitivities to food dyes of which those clients were previously unaware. Symptoms of such sensitivities are so varied that it can be difficult to identify food dyes as the culprit because many foods have added colour. Labeling laws in Canada have yet to require listing the specific food dye. Food labels will simply read, "colour."

Artificial Flavours

Aspartame, one of the most common artificial sweetening chemicals, has equally vehement supporters and opponents. The manufacturer and several government agencies support it as a sugar substitute, stating that it is perfectly safe. Doctors, both alternative (Janet Starr-Hull, ND) and medical (Russell Blaylock, MD), present evidence that aspartame is a poison that is slowly killing us. One ingredient in aspartame is wood alcohol, or methanol. Methanol is itself a poison, but once in the digestive system, it can break down into another poison, formaldehyde, which is in the same class as cyanide and arsenic—the only difference is that it is slow acting. Aspartame's primary target is the nervous system.[14]

Scientific findings on the health effects of aspartame are variable. Independent studies repeatedly find that this chemical causes nerve damage—the most common damage is to vision. Depending on the amount consumed, damage can be acute or slowly develop over a lifetime. There is evidence that aspartame poisoning can mimic several diseases, including fibromyalgia, multiple sclerosis, Alzheimer's, and lupus. Holisticmed.com reports that aspartame may be deadly for diabetics.[15] Meanwhile, some research finds no negative health effects from the sweetener. On its website, the manufacturer of aspartame cites studies showing that it is safe.[16] However, anti-aspartame groups contend that these corporately funded studies skew their findings to support the continued use of the artificial sweetener. Another aspartame promoter, the Calorie Control Council, presents itself as an independent organization, while its purpose is to represent the manufacturers and suppliers of alternative sweeteners.[17]

The official stance in the United States and Canada is that aspartame is safe for everyone except those who with phenylketonuria (PKU), a genetic disorder in which the body cannot process part of a protein called phenylalanine. The acceptable daily intake, according to Health Canada, is 40 mg per kilogram of body weight per day or the equivalent of eleven cans of diet soft drinks.[18] I cannot think of anyone who would consider it healthy to drink that many diet soft drinks in one day.

Approved in 1982 as a food additive, you will find this artificial sweetener in diet soft drinks, sugarless gum, yogurt, and diet foods. In recent years, I have noticed some reduction in its use by food companies.

Self-Help Tip: If you consume aspartame regularly and you have physical, visual, or mental problems, take the "60 day no-aspartame test."[19] If this chemical is affecting you, it can take as long as 60 days without this artificial sweetener to see any change in your symptoms.

Monosodium Glutamate (MSG) is an additive that can be described as "natural," depending on your point of view. MSG is a great flavour enhancer. It originated in Asia and then it was eagerly embraced in North America by manufacturers who wanted to make their processed foods taste better than competitive brands. Dr. Russell Blaylock provides scientific evidence that MSG promotes "cell death" in our bodies and that children are particularly sensitive. Long-term exposure can cause behaviour disorders, reproductive problems, obesity, and stunted growth. Regulating bodies allowed MSG in baby food from the 1940s until it was removed in 1969.[20] The most common symptom of overexposure to MSG is headache, but I have reports from clients of asthma attacks and chest pains. I have determined, through bioenergetic testing, that many of my clients are sensitive to MSG, which heightens symptoms and ill effects. Once MSG is out of their diet, unwanted symptoms are gone or dramatically reduced.

Found in a whole host of foods, MSG is difficult to avoid because it is also referred to by other names, such as hydrolyzed vegetable protein, autolyzed yeast, hydrolyzed yeast, spices, and vegetable powder. In the book *In Bad Taste: The MSG Syndrome*, Dr. George Schwarz reveals that the term "natural flavours" could, in fact mean MSG;[21] there is no way to be sure. Food served in restaurants may contain MSG originating from a spice or sauce used in the cooking process.

Preservatives

There are several preservatives with adverse health effects. The four of most concern to me are **BHT and BHA, TBHQ, Nitrate**, and **Sulfite**.

Butylated Hydroxytoluene (BHT) is a preservative added to a variety of foods in North America, despite reports of adverse health effects. It can affect the nervous system to the point of triggering behavioural problems and may be a problem for asthmatics. Environmentalist David Suzuki reports that long-term exposure to BHT has several adverse effects: inhibiting growth, allergic reactions in the skin, weight loss, damage to the liver and kidneys, blindness, reproductive problems, elevated blood cholesterol levels, and cancer. BHT can accumulate in fat tissue, which means the effects may take years to develop. England has banned BHT over concerns about its effects on children's health.[22]

A common use of BHT is in the packaging of cereal and crackers to maintain their freshness. This preservative may also be in frozen dinners, fruit drinks, margarine, chewing gum, and some fats and oils.

Butylated hydroxyanisole (BHA) is a derivative of BHT with similar risks. The International Agency for Research on Cancer classifies BHA as a possible human carcinogen. The European Commission on Endocrine Disruption has also listed BHA as a Category 1 priority substance, based on evidence that it interferes with hormone function. The use of both BHT and BHA is unrestricted in Canada.[23]

Tertiary Butyl hydroquinone (TBHQ) is a preservative that may affect health in sensitive individuals. The General Standard for Food Additives (GSFA) has set maximum limits for this preservative because of concerns about its health effects.[24] Health activist Shona Botes reports that overexposure to TBHQ may trigger these conditions in children: hyperactivity, asthma, rhinitis, and dermatitis.[25] However, based on studies with lab animals, the European Food Safety Association assigns little health risk to TBHQ.[26] Despite such assurances, some people have negatives reactions. My nephew, who has Pervasive Developmental Delay, becomes very agitated after exposure to TBHQ. Food processors use it to preserve foods such as fats, oils, frozen fish, crackers, crisps, and fast foods. It is also used in cosmetics, baby skin-care products, varnish, lacquers, and resins. Because there are no official limits on the use of TBHQ, the potential for harm is present with too much exposure; it is wise to limit intake from food and personal care products.

Nitrate as *sodium nitrate* is used to preserve meat to prevent botulism but not with some effects on human health. Once in the body, nitrate can produce nitrite, so the two terms are used interchangeably. In 1962, the World Health Organization established upper limits of nitrates in food and water after some studies linked long-term intake of nitrates to increased risk of cancer. However, debate over the safety of nitrates continues, and it continues to be the subject of research.[27] On its website, the Mayo Clinic warns that sodium nitrate can increase the risk of cardiovascular disease. Regulating bodies in both Canada and the United States express concerns about the health effects of nitrates. Health Canada points to ill effects on the thyroid from nitrates in drinking water and has established a maximum acceptable concentration at 45 mg nitrate per litre of water. They also report findings of considerably higher levels than this in vegetables in Canada, no doubt due to nitrogen-based fertilizers.[28] In the United States, the Food and Drug Administration (FDA) limits the levels of nitrates in processed foods to the minimum needed to prevent botulism. Among my clientele, many are sensitive to nitrates in food, making their reaction a more serious threat to health.

Sodium nitrate is found in cold cuts, bacon, hot dogs, beer, vegetables grown with chemical fertilizers, and in tap water. Heating or cooking meat containing nitrates (e.g., bacon) will cause carcinogenic compounds to form. Most meats sold at a deli counter will contain this preservative.

Sulphite (alternate spelling sulfite) is another class of preservative that keeps food from turning brown. This additive is also potentially harmful to asthmatics and those with allergies. Sulphites make the "ten priority food allergens" list reported by Health Canada. They give this warning: "some sulphite-sensitive people, many of whom also have asthma, may react to sulphites with allergy-like symptoms."[29] Dried fruits and fruit snacks are a common source; without this preservative, dried apricots are an unappetizing brown colour. Other sources include citrus drinks, many frozen items, such as potato products and TV dinners, red wine, and beer. Restaurant meals contain high amounts. Several medications contain sulphites such as blood pressure medications, steroids, antibiotics, pain relievers, and muscle relaxants. There are various forms: sodium bisulphite, sodium metabisulphite, potassium metabisulphite, sulfur dioxide, sodium sulphite, potassium sulphate, and bisulphate.

Refined foods and food additives represent human efforts to improve on the natural properties of food—enhancing taste, appearance, and extending shelf life. Unfortunately, these improvements may not extend our "shelf life" by triggering several negative health effects. Other forces influence our food choices that do not always serve us well. In Chapter 3, I examine how nutrition research, food marketing, and politics influence our concept of which foods are healthy.

Chapter Notes

1. Rudolph Ballantyne, MD, *Diet and Nutrition: A Holistic Approach* (Honesdale, Pennsylvania: The Himalayan International Institute, 1978), 20.

2. Lee Warren, BA, DD, "Is the Standard American Diet (SAD) Causing a Health Crisis? Part One," *PLIM REPORT,* 9, no.2 (2000), accessed April 2, 2014, www.plim.org/SAD.htm.

3. United States, Select Committee on Nutrition and Human Needs, "Dietary Goals for the United States" (1977): 2, accessed October 30, 2014, http://zerodisease.com/archive/Dietary_Goals_For_The_United_States.pdf.

4. Canada, Statistics Canada, "Canada spending more eating out," *Canada Year Book Overview 2006, Service Industries* (June 28, 2006, archived), accessed September 29, 2014, www41.statcan.ca/2006/0163/ceb0163_002-eng.htm.

5. *Super Size Me,* DVD, Directed by Morgan Spurlock (New York, New York: Kathbur Pictures/Studio on the Hudson, 2004).

6. James Balch and Phyllis Balch. *Prescription for Nutritional Healing,* Second edition (Garden City Park, New York: Avery Publishing, 1997, 14-17).

7. Robert H. Lustig, MD, MSL, *Fat Chance: Beating the Odds against Sugar, Processed Foods, Obesity and Disease* (New York, New York: Hudson Street Press, Penguin Group, 2013), 4.

8. Michael Pollan, *In Defense of Food: An Eater's Manifesto* (New York, New York: Penguin Press, 2008), 112.

9. Robert H. Lustig, *Fat Chance,* 166-9.

10. Miriam E. Bocarsly, et al., "High-fructose corn syrup causes characteristics of obesity in rats: Increased body weight, body fat and triglyceride levels," *Pharmacology Biochemistry and Behavior,* 97 no. 1 (November 2010): 101-106, accessed November 2, 2014, http://www.sciencedirect.com/science/article/pii/S0091305710000614.

11. Dana Flavin, "Metabolic Danger of High-Fructose Corn Syrup," *Life Extension Magazine* (December 2008), accessed May 20, 2014, http://www.lef.org/magazine/mag2008/dec2008_Metabolic-Dangers-of-High-Fructose-Corn-Syrup_01.htm.

12. Janet Starr-Hull, ND, "Food Additives to Avoid," *Sweetpoison.com,* accessed May 21, 2014, www.sweetpoison.com/food-additives-to-avoid.html.

13. Karen Lau, et al., "Synergistic Interactions between Commonly Used Food Additives in a Developmental Neurotoxicity Test," *Toxicological Sciences* 9 no.1 (March 2006): 178-187, accessed May 21, 2014, http://www.ncbi.nlm.nih.gov/pubmed/16352620.

14. Russell L. Blaylock, MD, *Excitotoxins: The Taste that Kills* (Albuquerque, New Mexico: Health Press NA, 1997).

15. "Aspartame Toxicity Info Center," *Holisticmed.com,* accessed September 10, 2013, http://www.holisticmed.com/aspartame/.

16. "Nutrasweet Deemed Safe by Expert Panel," *Nutrasweet.com,* accessed September 12, 2014, http://www.nutrasweet.com/media/aspar001.pdf.

17. "Aspartame Information Center," *Calorie Control Council, Aspartame.org,* accessed September 12, 2014, www.aspartame.org.

18. Canada, Health Canada, "The Safety of Sugar Substitutes," last modified April 30, 2008, http://www.hc-sc.gc.ca/hl-vs/iyh-vsv/food-aliment/sugar_sub_sucre-eng.php.

19. "Aspartame Toxicity Info Center," *Holisticmed.com.*

20. Russell L. Blaylock, *Excitotoxins,* 33-37.

21. George R. Schwarz, MD, *In Bad Taste: The MSG Syndrome* (Santa Fe, New Mexico: Health Press, 1988).

22. "BHA and BHT," *David Suzuki Foundation, davidsuzuki.org,* accessed June 14, 2014, www.davidsuzuki.org/issues/health/science/toxics/chemicals-in-your-cosmetics---bha-and-bhti/.

23. Ibid.

24. "Evaluation of National Assessment of Intake of tert-Butylhydroquinone (TBHQ)," Prepared by the Fifty-first meeting of the Joint FAO/WHO, Expert Committee on Food Additives (JECFA), *International Programme on Chemical Safety* (1999), accessed November 12, 2014, ttp://www.inchem.org/documents/jecfa/jecmono/v042je26.htm.

25. Shona Botes, "TBHQ: Why This Preservative Should Be Avoided," *Natural News* (February 14, 2011), accessed June 15, 2014, http://www.naturalnews.com/031318_TBHQ_food_preservatives.html.

26. R. Anton et al., "Opinion of the Scientific Panel on Food Additives, Flavourings, Processing Aids and Materials in Contact with Food on a request from the Commission related to tertiary-Butylhydroquinone (TBHQ)," *The EFSA Journal* 84 (2004): 1-50, accessed November 12, 2014, http://www.efsa.europa.eu/en/efsajournal/doc/84.pdf.

27. Martijn Katan, "Nitrates in Food: Harmful or Healthy?" *American Journal of Clinical Nutrition* 90 no.1 (July 2009): 11-12, accessed June 15, 2014, doi: 10.3945/ajcn.2009.28014.

28. Canada, Health Canada, "Guidelines for Canadian Drinking Water Quality: Guideline Technical Document—Nitrate and Nitrite" (June 2013), last modified August 27, 2014, http://www.hc-sc.gc.ca/ewh-semt/pubs/water-eau/nitrate_nitrite/index-eng.php.

29. Canada, Health Canada, "Sulphites – One of the top ten priority food allergens," last modified October 26, 2012, http://www.hc-sc.gc.ca/fn-an/pubs/securit/2012-allergen_sulphites-sulfites/index-eng.php.

3: POLITICS IN RESEARCH AND MARKETING

Decisions about which foods are health-promoting are fraught with controversy. That nutrition science is only 100 years old has something to do with this. Research methods used to study our relationship with food do not always prove reliable. Food production has become a big business, and as a result, economics and politics influence what is generally accepted as healthy food. Consumers must sift through the mixed messages from governments, health organizations, and food companies. To make dietary choices that are health supportive, it is imperative to understand the politics of nutrition research and food marketing.

Nutrition Research

The human diet includes a wide variety of foods that all work together to impact our health. Yet most nutrition research focuses on one food or one nutrient as if it could be of benefit apart from other foods and nutrients. This is a well-respected research method—isolate one factor so you can study it. However, this does not work well to explain our dietary relationships because of many nutrients working in various combinations. Marion Nestle, a New York University nutritionist, is quoted as saying: "The problem with nutrient-by-nutrient nutrition science is that it takes the nutrient out of the context of the food, the food out of the context of the diet, and the diet out of the context of the lifestyle."[1]

An understanding of nutrition research helps us make educated decisions about what to believe. Studies of nutrition in relation to human health take one of several forms: long-term population studies, animal research, double-blind controlled studies, and comparative population studies. Whatever the research method used, there are limitations to its reliability.

Population studies track the diet of a society, group, or subgroup (e.g., women, men), typically over time, and then compare their health outcomes. Because large populations are involved, one would expect the results to be more reliable. However, the key to this method is reliable tracking of dietary habits and controlling for other factors that affect health—genetics, environment, age, lifestyle, etc. One of the most famous population studies tracking the effects of diet on health, the Women's Health Study,[2] relied on self-reported dietary habits, which the authors admitted later participants routinely misreported.[3] Think about it! At the end of the day, could you name exactly what you ate, and the quantity consumed?

Animal research with mice or rats is common because these subjects are more affordable and manageable. The animals' life spans are shorter, making any nutritional effects show up faster. In animal studies, one food is typically studied in an artificial environment in which the animals are fed only that food. This does not relate well to humans, whose diets and lifestyles are never this limited or controlled. Generalizing results from animals to humans is the primary drawback of this research method.

Researchers consider the "randomized double-blind study" as the gold standard of study methods. There is a study group and a control group whose diets differ in one specific way. To eliminate bias during the study neither the researchers nor the participants know which group is which. This method is often used in animal studies, because, as already noted, it is easy to control their diet, and they are not aware of any diet differences. With human subjects, there are practical and ethical problems in double-blind studies. Objectivity is almost impossible to achieve with human participants because we recognize food by taste and appearance and often have opinions about the health of certain foods (e.g., sugary treats). In addition, there is the ethical dilemma of denying humans nutrients. In the book, *Healing Cancer: Complementary Vitamin & Drug Treatments*, highly respected nutrition researchers Dr. Abram Hoffer and Linus Pauling recognized this and proposed using natural control groups—those who decide on their own not to participate after initially agreeing to serve as study subjects. Their decision to drop out takes the onus off the researchers' denial of a food or nutrient.[4] Unfortunately, nutrition researchers have not embraced the natural control group method. The double-blind study is practical only in nutrition research involving lab animals, the limitations of which are discussed in the previous paragraph.

Comparative population research examines the typical diets of different cultural or geographic areas in relation to the health trends in those populations. Such studies are purely observational; there is no information gathered from individuals. It is unfortunate that sometimes the data from these studies are oversimplified. For example, comparative studies found the Japanese ate a lot of soy *and* had low rates of heart disease. North Americans did not eat as much soy, but had high rate of heart disease. As a result, North American nutrition guidelines deemed soy as a heart-healthy food and heavily marketed it as such. However, soy foods were adopted out of context with the Japanese diet culture. This has produced unintended ill effects (more on this in Chapter 4). There is also the French paradox. The French have, on average, lower rates of cardiovascular disease than North Americans do. As a result, the typical French diet has become the source of much attention. Their diets are high in fat and red wine. For some, this led to justifying diets high in fat and red wine, which may or may not be valid. The China Study researchers, who used the comparative population approach, admit to the challenges in making definitive conclusions about diet and health, stating, "Establishing proof for any one factor and any one disease is nearly impossible."[5] Evidence that X illness happens more often when X food is eaten does not mean that the food *causes* the illness. It is *possible* the food is *associated* with the illness, but there might be other factors.

The following story illustrates how an association can be misinterpreted as a causal relationship. A person went into a health store and noticed that all the people there were older and had health problems. That evening, the same person went to a nightclub where the patrons, who were drinking and smoking heavily, were all young and healthy looking. Based on the evidence, the observer concluded that health stores are bad for your health, while going to bars will keep you young and healthy. This may sound like a silly conclusion, but it is not far removed from some conclusions in nutrition research. An association of events is often mistakenly viewed as cause and effect.

An unfortunate reality is that food companies sponsor most nutrition research with a vested interest in the outcome. In his book, *In Defense of Food: An Eater's Manifesto,* Michael Pollan maintains that such research is more likely to produce findings favourable to that industry's products—processed foods.[6] The research that we hear about is also filtered because of who controls medical and scientific journals. Journals may receive funding from the food industry so studies challenging the interests of large food companies may never be published.[7]

Because of the complexities of the human diet, proving cause and effect in nutrition research is extremely difficult. In addition, there are other factors affecting health—lifestyle, environment, emotional health, and cultural norms—that have nothing to do with diet. Whatever the research method used, it is difficult to make *definitive* claims about how specific foods affect human health, in particular across different cultures. General claims of benefit are possible, but always in the context of other factors that affect health. Nevertheless, food manufacturers, government agencies, and health organizations make health-related claims about food and food products all the time.

Food Guide Follies

Health Canada's current Food Guide may result from flawed nutrition research and influence from powerful food lobbies. In developing "food guides," governments consult with food marketing boards, which are influenced by the food industry. In an exposé of such influence in the United States, Marion Nestle reveals how adept food companies are at obtaining support for their products from both governments and professional health organizations.[8] Voicing similar concerns are the researchers/authors of the China Study, who claim that the National Institutes of Health (U.S.) is strongly influenced by the meat, dairy, and egg industries.[9] Economic realities are no doubt at play. Governments are apt to listen to food marketing boards and big corporations because they are a critical part of the country's economy. I believe such political influence is why many people, even so-called experts, continue to deem margarine part of a "healthy diet," even after considerable evidence to contrary. (More on this in Chapter 4)

Food Marketing

Food production and processing is big business, but what is good for business is not always good for consumers. With respect to food, the capitalist system demonstrates its weakness: the most profit is made from food "products" that can be branded. Brand preferences drive food industry profits and, to be competitive, foods must taste, smell, or look better than the other brands. Whole foods are difficult to brand. Not much can be done to distinguish one broccoli bunch from another. Therefore, the competitive edge in the food business will always involve foods that are processed (i.e., food in boxes, bags, and cans) because manufacturers can add or remove ingredients to set them apart from other food products.

In a free-market economy, most of the information we receive about food and its benefits comes from food manufacturers, rather than government or non-profit organizations. The reason is simple: Unlike governments and non-profits, both manufacturers of processed food and food marketing boards can afford expensive advertising for their food products. This leaves the consumer at the mercy of slick marketing campaigns. Food manufacturers have historically marketed to consumers by catering to their taste buds, but more recently, there have been clever appeals to consumers' concerns about health. Slogans make foods appear more nutritious than they are, e.g., "all natural," or "low fat." I have noticed that marketing can even appeal to consumers' awareness of food components now known to be beneficial. For example, manufacturers are adding omega-3 fatty acids and probiotics to products and marketing them as health promoting, even though these fragile substances may not survive processing or storage on grocery shelves.

Many people turn to non-profit organizations for objective advice, but any organization can be co-opted. Michael Pollan uncovered one such example. In his book *In Defense of Food*, he states: "The American Heart Association currently bestows (for a fee) its *heart healthy* seal of approval on Lucky Charms™, Cocoa Puffs™, and Trix cereals™, Yoo-hoo lite™ chocolate drink, and Healthy Choice's Premium Caramel Swirl Ice Cream Sandwich™."[10] I doubt anyone would believe these products, which are full of sugar, preservatives, and processed fats, to be heart healthy. In Canada, the Heart and Stroke Foundation has received funding for its marketing campaigns from the manufacturer of a popular brand of margarine. Is it coincidence that the Foundation proclaims margarine to be "heart healthy?"

You would think that organizations representing dieticians would be reliable sources of information. Think again! The governing body of registered dieticians in the United States receives funding from the food industry. In her book, *Food Politics: How the Food Industry Influences Nutrition and Health,* Marion Nestle makes the case that industry funding is affecting dieticians' nutritional advice. She states, "Indeed the American Dietetic Association's [now the Academy of Nutrition and Dietetics] stance on dietary advice is firmly pro-industry; one of its basic tenets is that there is no such thing as a bad food."[11] I have heard a similar statement from Canadian dieticians, e.g., "there are no bad foods, only bad portions." As a holistic nutritionist in private practice with no business affiliations, I do not have to hedge my position—there are definitely foods that are bad for our health.

In Canada, there is the Canadian Digestive Health Foundation, a charitable organization established in 2007 by the Canadian Association of Gastroenterology. Its mission is "to reduce suffering and improve quality of life by providing trusted, accessible, and accurate information about digestive health and disease." The name of the organization, its founder, and purpose would lead most people to think this is an independent, neutral body. However, the priority partners listed on its website in 2013 included two well-known yogurt manufacturers and two pharmaceutical companies.[12] One TV commercial for a brand of yogurt mentioned this foundation.

Our beliefs about which foods are healthy are based on three powerful influences: 1) Nutrition research that may or may not be accurate, 2) the profit interests of corporations, organizations, and government, and 3) media spin. It is critical to be aware of who is behind any report about food's influence on health. Be wary of accepting each new study's findings as irrefutable. Unless you are trained in nutrition and in analyzing research methods, it will be difficult to know which studies to believe. The best studies consider multiple factors and make links and associations, instead of generalizations that make big news. Researchers who publish studies are required to list their affiliations, which is apt to influence the interpretation of findings. Health organizations also have affiliations that must be considered before we accept their "seals of approval." If we only listen to the media reports about nutrition research, we are subject to political and economic agendas and the goal to attract and wow viewers/readers. Food marketing messages must always be taken with a grain of salt.

Throughout this book, I refer to numerous studies and experts' opinions, and try to ensure these sources are reliable. I also include studies that may be flawed but also explain why I question their findings. Integrity in nutrition research and diet guidelines is possible; otherwise, no book on nutrition has value. However, it is also critical to understand that nutrition is a new field of research. New research discoveries may disprove last year's nutrition "facts." It is little wonder that there are misconceptions about the health of some foods. In the next chapter, I discuss several foods widely accepted as healthy that are far from it.

Chapter Notes

1. Marion Nestle, as quoted by Michael Pollan, *In Defense of Food: An Eater's Manifesto* (New York, New York: Penguin Press, 2008), 62.

2. Julie E. Buring, ScD and I-Min Lee, MD, ScD, "Study Design," Women's Health Study, Harvard Medical School and Brigham and Women's Hospital, accessed November 17, 2014, http://whs.bwh.harvard.edu/methods.html.

3. "Low-Fat Diet Not a Cure-All," *Harvard School of Public Health, The Nutrition Source, Hsph.harvard.edu,* accessed November 17, 2014, http://www.hsph.harvard.edu/nutritionsource/low-fat/.

4. Abram Hoffer, MD, FRCP with Linus Pauling, PhD, *Healing Cancer: Complementary Vitamin and Drug Treatments* (Toronto, Ontario: Canadian College of Naturopathic Medicine Press, 2004).

5. Colin T. Campbell, PhD, and Thomas M. Campbell II, *The China Study: Startling Implications for Diet, Weight Loss and Long-Term Health* (Dallas, Texas: Benbella Books, 2006), 38.

6. Michael Pollan, *In Defense of Food: An Eater's Manifesto,* 34.

7. Marion Nestle, *Food Politics: How the Food Industry Influences Nutrition and Health* (University of California Press, 2007).

8. Ibid.

9. Colin T. Campbell, PhD., and Thomas M. Campbell II, *The China Study.*

10. Michael Pollan, *In Defense of Food,* 156.

11. Marion Nestle, *Food Politics,* 127-8.

12. Since my initial research on The Canadian Digestive Health Foundation, the website changed. It appears the foundation has distanced itself from commercial interests. As of November 17, 2014, the website lists an affiliation with one pharmaceutical whose role was to assist with marketing. http://www.cdhf.ca/bank/document_en/84the-evolution-of-the-cdhf.pdf#zoom=100.

4: FOOD MYTHS DEBUNKED

Health-conscious consumers are apt to hear conflicting information about several foods and food groups. As explained in Chapter 3, nutrition research, economic interests, politics, and media spin have combined to influence our beliefs about food. As a result, there are misconceptions about certain foods and their role in health. Even after there is evidence to the contrary, the original belief about these foods continues and enters the realm of myth. In this chapter, I reveal six food myths that, if not debunked, could negatively affect your health. These myths involve cow's milk as the perfect food; milk as a source of calcium; the role of saturated fats in heart disease; eggs and cholesterol; the proposed health benefits of soy; and grains as a dietary staple.

Milk: "Nature's Perfect Food"?

Myth: Cow's milk and milk products (cheese, yogurt) are a dietary necessity for humans throughout their lives.

Fact: Not only do some people not tolerate cow's milk and its products, but there are also health concerns for anyone consuming them after weaning.

Here are some interesting *facts* about milk:

- Cow's milk *is* a perfect food—for calves—but only until they are weaned.
- Humans are the only species that drinks milk past weaning.
- Humans are the only species that drinks the milk of another species.
- Much of the world's population does not drink milk into adulthood.
- The National Dairy Council estimates that 25 percent of the North American population is intolerant to lactose in milk.[1]
- The ability to produce lactase, the enzyme needed to digest milk into adulthood, was an evolutionary development among animal herders in Eastern Europe starting approximately 7,500 years ago. A 2009 study suggests that this genetic development persists among Eastern Europeans, making them better able to digest milk products than people originating in other regions.[2]

Much of this information about cow's milk is common knowledge, yet government "food guides" in both the United States and Canada still consider dairy foods as a separate food group. The only concession in these guides is the allowance for "milk alternatives," from sources such as soy. A Milk Marketing Board in Canada advertises the purported health benefits of drinking milk. Its latest advertising slogan poses the question, "are you getting enough?"

The most serious concern about cow's milk is its nutritional suitability for human infants. Since the late 1800s, infant formula from cow's milk has been touted as being equal to, or better than, human milk. This message continues, even after nutritional science learned that the ratio of proteins, carbohydrates, and fats in cow's milk differs from human milk. Human milk is lower in protein and higher in carbohydrates than cow's milk. Breast-fed babies receive key immune support from their mothers that cow's milk formula cannot duplicate. Attempts to fortify these formulas with missing nutrients (omega-3's, vitamins, and probiotics) are laudable, but as health education specialist Annemarie Colbin emphasizes, the ratio of fat, protein, and carbohydrates cannot be adjusted to match mother's milk.[3]

Modern dairy products undergo processes intended to make them safer, but unfortunately reduce their health benefits. Pasteurization was introduced in the 1890s to reduce the risk of highly contagious bacterial diseases, including bovine tuberculosis and brucellosis, from being transmitted through raw milk. There are other risks, including E. coli, Listeria, and Salmonella. It all comes down to how hygienic the dairy farm is. While pasteurization kills bacteria in the milk, it also kills beneficial enzymes that would make milk nutritious (at least for those who can tolerate it). In Canada, it is illegal to sell raw milk, but cheese made from raw milk is allowed, because making the cheese destroys harmful bacteria. In France, raw milk cheese is considered the standard for high-quality cheese. Some European countries also allow the sale of raw milk.

Homogenization is another process introduced for mostly esthetic reasons. In this process, the fat particles (cream) fracture so they stay in suspension in the milk, rather than rising to the top. Unfortunately, fracturing fat particles increases their rate of rancidity and oxidation, both of which damage the fat and make the milk hazardous to health. There is also the risk that our bodies cannot digest the "fractured" milk fat. Nutrition researcher Mary Enig presents evidence that homogenization may contribute to the increase in allergies to milk.[4]

There are several potential health risks from drinking cow's milk. Some people have lactose intolerance—the inability to digest the milk sugar lactose. They may experience a variety of digestive problems and impaired immunity. Others are merely sensitive to dairy and have only mild discomfort. Exposure to bovine estrogen in the milk also has the potential to affect human hormone balance. Studies of large populations have linked dairy consumption to juvenile diabetes, insulin resistance, heart disease, Crohn's disease, prostate cancer, premature puberty, and multiple sclerosis. Based on considerable research on the health effects of milk, Dr. Neal Barnard has concluded that avoiding early childhood exposure to cow's milk could reduce the risk of type 1 diabetes.[5]

My clinical experience is that many people do not thrive on milk. In my years of testing for food sensitivities, the most common one detected is to cow's milk and its products. While consuming milk, my clients with a dairy sensitivity experienced one or more of these health issues: frequent colds, sinus congestion, allergies, lung congestion, acne, eczema, constipation, diarrhea, joint pain, edema, and overweight.

Eliminating milk invariably eliminated or reduced their health concerns. I, too, have a history of issues with milk:

> I attribute some of my health problems to drinking cow's milk from infancy into early adulthood. As a baby, I was fed evaporated cow's milk because my mother believed the doctor's assurance that it was just as good as breast milk. While still at the hospital (nine days), I cried so much the staff assumed I was hungry. They began feeding me infant cereal (*Pablum*) before I left the hospital, which was likely another challenge to my digestive system. Through infancy and childhood, I suffered from both diarrhea and constipation. I had many colds and, at age 8, I had pleurisy. In my teens, acne was very problematic and the frequent colds continued. Years later, while training in holistic nutrition, I realized that all these issues were because of my milk intolerance. Did I have this from the start or was it because I had cow's milk as an infant? Perhaps another factor was the introduction of solid foods too early. I will never know for sure, but I know that after eliminating milk, my colds were less frequent, my sinuses were less congested, my skin cleared, and bowel regularity improved.

It is imperative to determine if you can tolerate milk and its products, but this is not always clear. Symptoms of intolerance vary widely. Your symptoms may differ from the ones I experienced. The process of identifying dairy intolerance is presented in Chapter 8. If you can consume milk products with ill effects, I still recommend your limit intake. Because of homogenization and pasteurization, milk is neither a perfect food nor without health risks. Chapter 7 provides my dietary guidelines for dairy consumption and dairy alternatives.

Calcium and Milk

Myth: Cow's milk is the best source of calcium.
Fact: Calcium in cow's milk is not easily absorbed.
Myth: If you stop drinking cow's milk, you will get osteoporosis.
Fact: There is no proof that drinking cow's milk prevents osteoporosis.

Despite the health warnings in the previous section, you may continue to consume cow's milk because of a belief that the calcium in milk builds bones and prevents osteoporosis. Yes, dairy foods are high in calcium, but we may not absorb enough to be of benefit. There is no convincing evidence that drinking milk makes strong bones. A 2005 study found that increasing intake of milk or other dairy products was not associated with promoting child and adolescent bone mineralization.[6] Research has even cast doubt on the belief that milk drinking prevents osteoporosis. In the Nurses' Health Study, involving 72,000 nurses tracked over many years, milk consumption was not associated with a lower risk of hip fracture, a measure of bone strength. In fact, women who drank milk twice a day were as likely to suffer a bone break as women who drank it once a week.[7]

According to a 2003 report from the World Health Organization (WHO), countries consuming the most milk products also have the highest rates of osteoporosis. The report's recommendations to prevent osteoporosis are based on several factors apart from milk, such as consumption of green vegetables and legumes, adequate vitamin D, a range of minerals, weight bearing exercise, and exposure to sunshine.[8] The message is clear: milk is not the only factor. However, over ten years after the WHO report, medical doctors, dieticians, and government health authorities continue to promote cow's milk as the primary source of calcium.

When I tell clients to stop drinking milk, the usual question is, "But how am I going to get my calcium?" I answer simply, "Eat your greens (green leafy vegetables, broccoli, Brussels sprouts), nuts (almonds), seeds (sesame, sunflower), canned fish (salmon, sardines), and legumes (chickpeas)." An additional advantage of these foods is that many contain other minerals—magnesium, boron, manganese, and vanadium—that are essential for supporting healthy bones. A holistic perspective also considers the body's ability to absorb these minerals from the diet. In Part 3, I outline the factors affecting mineral absorption.

Saturated Fats and Heart Disease

Myth: Saturated fats are the cause of heart disease.
Fact: The health risks attributed to saturated fats are based on flawed research. Several factors contribute to the development of heart disease.

Humans have been eating saturated fats for millennia with little concern. In the 1940s, research identified saturated fats as a major health risk for cardiovascular disease and cancer. By the 1990s, some nutritionists challenged this position when they realized there were flaws in the early research on saturated fats. In their book *Nourishing Traditions: The Cookbook that Challenges Politically Correct Nutrition and the Diet Dictocrats,* Sally Fallon and Mary Enig reveal: "...the fats used were hydrogenated fats although the results were presented as though the culprit was saturated fats."[9] Researchers had used coconut oil and palm oil, both saturated fats, but in a hydrogenated form, which we now know produces unhealthy *trans fats.* Some years ago, food manufacturers developed hydrogenation to preserve fats so they would not spoil too quickly. Processed foods containing hydrogenated fats (i.e., trans fats) have a longer shelf life, but, as outlined in Chapter 2, eating such foods may shorten our *shelf life.*

Knowledge of the health risks of trans fats did not surface until the late 1990s. Around the same time, there was some rethinking of the position on saturated fats. A 2001 review of all the research to that point made this conclusion: "the low-fat campaign has been based on little scientific evidence and may have caused unintended health consequences...Only one study has ever found a significant positive association between saturated fat intake and risk of cardiovascular disease."[10]

Meanwhile, for over 30 years, government health organizations have told us to limit intake of saturated fat to prevent cardiovascular disease. Instead, we were advised to use polyunsaturated fats from sources such as sunflower, canola, corn, safflower, soy. Many of us discarded beef lard in favour of vegetable oils for frying and deep-frying. The "healthy" spread became margarine made from vegetable oils instead of butter. Unfortunately, we reduced our intake of saturated fats, only to replace them with foods containing damaging trans fats. Fallon and Enig give us this warning: "Consumption of hydrogenated fats is associated with a host of serious diseases, not only cancer but also atherosclerosis, diabetes, obesity, immune system dysfunction, low birth-weight babies, birth defects, decreased visual acuity, sterility, difficulty in lactation and problems with bones and tendons."[11]

Since reducing our intake of saturated fats, we have seen dramatic increases in the rate of heart disease and its major risk factor, obesity. In his book *Feed Your Brain, Lose Your Belly*, brain surgeon Larry McCleary comments on this issue, stating, "Adult obesity and overweight statistics have increased by about 50 percent since the Dietary Goals [to lower saturated fat] were announced [by the federal government, in 1977]. That bears repeating: a 50 percent increase in obesity/overweight correlated with a 10 percent decrease in fat content in the diet."[12] While these events are associated and not necessarily proof, that trans fats are the cause, most holistic nutritionists believe in the correlation between obesity and consumption of processed foods that contain trans fats. We have blamed saturated fats for our health problems when the real culprit has been trans fats.

Efforts to reduce trans fats in the food supply may not be enough to make a difference. In 2002, Health Canada required all food labels to list the trans fat content. In 2009, the Trans Fat Task Force in Canada recommended limits, but still not elimination of the artificial fat from the food supply. They allowed a trans fat content of 2 percent of total fat content in margarines and 5 percent in other food products, except meat and dairy products. Canadian researcher and nutrition author Udo Erasmus, PhD, warns that, unfortunately, no amount of trans fat is safe.[13] Government "limits" on trans fats leave the onus on consumers to read labels and, by their choices, eventually force trans fats out of the food supply. Unfortunately, not everyone is concerned enough to avoid foods and snacks that contain these dangerous fats. In 2010, the Canadian Heart and Stroke Foundation stated that Canada "urgently needs trans fat regulation" after making this startling discovery: "The bakery sector in particular, including between 33% and 75% of some of these products, continues to be riddled with unnecessarily high levels of trans fats."[14]

Food processing can damage fats in other ways. Fats and oils are highly susceptible to damage from exposure to heat and light, which both happen during food processing. Most of the cooking oils and salad dressings sold in supermarkets contain oils that are extracted from their source (usually seeds) using high heat. Udo Erasmus warns that this heat extraction process damages the fats and oils, making them rancid and an additional threat to good health.[15] I take exception to Canada's Food Guide because it lists vegetable oils as a source of healthy fats. Most of these oils are damaged goods.

The creation of margarine is a prime example of destroying the nutritional value of oils and, in the process, our own health. During the Depression and Second World War, there was a shortage of butter, and margarine filled the void. After the war, margarine producers wanted to keep their customers. Because of misinterpreted research that demeaned saturated fats, manufacturers convinced us that margarine was "better than butter." Of course, these early margarines were hydrogenated because at that time, this process was the only way to keep vegetable oils solid. When, in the 1990s, research found hydrogenation to be a source of trans fats, manufacturers of margarine changed their production methods; this allowed the marketing of margarine as "trans fat free." The problem is that turning liquid oil into a solid still requires considerable processing. The oils that go into margarine are already rancid (i.e., damaged) from the high heat used to extract oil from the seeds (e.g., canola, soy, corn). The manufacturing process for margarine, outlined by Sally Fallon, should turn anyone's stomach:

- Oil is subjected to hydrogen gas in a high-pressure, high-temperature reactor
- Addition of soap-like emulsifiers and starch to improve consistency
- Steam cleaning at high temperatures
- Bleaching to make the colour more appetizing
- Dying and flavouring to make it resemble butter.[16]

The resulting product is neither natural nor healthy. Unfortunately, some trusted health organizations and professional associations continue to promote margarine as "heart healthy." I wonder how long this misconception will continue, and how the public will react when they learn the facts about it.

Other fat-containing foods were given a bad rap because of fears about dietary fat. For a time, people avoided eating nuts because of their fat content. Then several studies linked the consumption of nuts with a decrease in the risk for cardiac disease.[17] While there are several nutritional benefits to nuts (protein, fibre, vitamins), we know they are a source of beneficial fats called *omega-3*s. These fats are lacking in the Standard American Diet. The 2001 review of research on fats, cited earlier in this section, concluded that while total dietary fat apparently has little bearing on the risk of heart disease, the ratio between types of fat does. The authors concluded that adding omega-3 fatty acids to the diet "substantially reduces coronary and total mortality" in heart patients. If omega-3s can do this for people who already had a heart attack, think what they could do to prevent it![18]

It is widely accepted that heart disease has other contributing factors apart from fats—undue stress, toxins (smoking), lack of exercise, and excess sugar. As revealed in Chapter 2, sugar intake in North America skyrocketed with the introduction of processed foods; this has coincided with a rapid rise in the rate of heart disease. John Yudkin, a British physiologist and nutritionist, was the first to make the connection between excess sugar and heart disease in the 1950s.[19] Fallon and Enig explain how this works: "Elevated triglycerides in the blood have been positively linked to proneness to heart disease, but these triglycerides do not come directly from dietary fats; they are made in the liver from any excess sugars that have not been used for energy."[20] The relationship between stress and heart disease is discussed in Chapter 6.

Eggs and Cholesterol

Myth: Eggs are high in cholesterol, so they must increase blood levels of cholesterol and the risk of heart disease.
Fact: Recent research shows no such correlation and, in fact, suggests that moderate consumption of eggs could lower blood cholesterol.

To understand how eggs were once vilified, we must consider the early research on cholesterol's role in human health. Studies in the 1950s linked high cholesterol levels in the blood to atherosclerosis and heart disease. Unfortunately, this research made a critical error in its conclusions. This is a case of a weak association being given a causal relationship. We now know more about how cholesterol works in the body. Cholesterol is a hormone that the body naturally produces in response to several factors. It is well established that only 10 to 20 percent of cholesterol comes from diet. Some people naturally manufacture more than others do, perhaps because of heredity. Cholesterol levels will also increase in response to damage to the lining of blood vessels from diet—trans fats, damaged fats, excess sugar, processed food— and lifestyle factors such as toxic exposure and physical and emotional stress. For cholesterol to be damaging, it must also be oxidized, which recent research showed to be related to the factors just mentioned.[21] In fact, cholesterol is the body's repair mechanism, applied like a patch over a wound, which in this case is damage to the arteries. The problem is that the "patch" becomes plaque that clogs the arteries and eventually triggers a stroke or heart attack. Clearly, the focus also needs to be on preventing damage to arteries, and not just on limiting cholesterol consumption.

There is now recognition in the medical community that cholesterol's role in cardiovascular disease is not as once thought. Cholesterol comes in two forms— LDL (low-density lipoprotein) and HDL (high-density lipoprotein). LDL triggers the formation of artery-clogging plaque, while HDL cholesterol is beneficial because it takes excess cholesterol out of circulation. A 2009 study tracking over 100,000 heart attack patients found only half had damaging LDL cholesterol levels that would have put them at risk for a cardiovascular event. However, most of those who had heart attacks had low levels of good HDL cholesterol. The study's researchers called for "better treatment" to increase the levels of HDL cholesterol.[22] There is a natural and effective "treatment" to increase HDL cholesterol; it is a health-supportive diet and lifestyle. This is not new information. In the 1980s, Dr. Dean Ornish determined through his clinical trials that diet and lifestyle changes were more effective in reducing the risk of heart attacks than cholesterol-lowering medications. However, Dr. Ornish's diet program also limited egg consumption.[23] That recommendation is now open to question.

While eggs are high in cholesterol, they are also high in lecithin, which helps break down the cholesterol. This means that we likely absorb very little of the cholesterol in eggs. The Harvard School of Public Health cites several studies that found increased egg consumption did *not* increase the risk of cardiovascular disease in either men or women. Egg consumers had lower serum cholesterol levels than those who abstained from eggs.[24] The myth that eggs increase damaging (LDL) cholesterol has been shattered. Unfortunately, some health authorities continue to advise against eggs, but I maintain that eating three to four eggs per week is beneficial for most people (except those with egg sensitivities), even those with high LDL cholesterol.

Soy: Not so Good

Myth: Soy is heart healthy, lowers cholesterol, and balances hormones.
Fact: There is limited evidence of these therapeutic benefits from soy and some risk from its over-consumption.

Soy has been a staple of the Asian diet for centuries. Some time ago, population studies revealed that rates of cardiovascular disease were lower in Asian countries. Researchers concluded that high soy consumption must protect the heart. As a result, soy became the new miracle health food in North America. In the rush to embrace soy, food companies gave little heed to the form in which Asians consumed it. Their dietary soy was almost exclusively fermented. In fact, Asians consider the unfermented soybean an inferior food.

There are nutritional concerns about unfermented soy. Nutrient analysis has established that soybeans contain phytates, which, when eaten in large amounts, can block the uptake of essential minerals such as calcium, magnesium, copper, iron, and especially zinc. A 2009 study at Iowa State University did not confirm a mineral-blocking action, but tracked soy intake and its effects for only 10 weeks.[25] I consider this too short a time to make definitive conclusions. Soy also contains oxalates, which, according to the American Chemical Society, can bind with calcium and increase risk for the development of kidney stones.[26] In *Nourishing Traditions*, Sally Fallon and Mary Enig maintain that soy can depress thyroid function.[27]

Fermentation of soy neutralizes the phytates and eliminates their mineral-blocking action. Fermented soy sources include miso, tempeh, natto, and soy sauce. Unfermented forms that contain phytates include tofu, bean curd, soy milk, protein powders, soy-based infant formula, and meat alternatives in vegetarian foods. In North America, food manufacturers routinely add soy protein isolate (unfermented) to processed foods—another reason to limit such "food". However, fermentation does not reduce the potential for ill effects on thyroid function.

A purported benefit of soy is the reduction of cholesterol. In the previous section, evidence was presented to question a single-minded focus on lowering cholesterol, but this connection needs to be addressed because soy products may make this claim. Joe Schwarcz, who holds a PhD in chemistry, questions the cholesterol-lowering benefits of soy. He states, "Some 22 clinical investigations have been carried out since 1999 examining the effect of large amounts of soy protein on cholesterol levels. The results have been unimpressive: cholesterol was lowered on average by just 3 percent."[28] Soy foods and soy-containing supplements are clearly not critical to lowering cholesterol.

Soy may promote hormone balance in some women under some circumstances. The phytoestrogens in soy can also upset hormone balance, but there is disagreement about the specific impact. Some say it is normalizing, while others say it is destabilizing. There may be a protective effect against breast cancer, but not for everyone. Long-term studies of Asians have indeed shown that soy intake is protective, but only if consumed early in life. It appears there are three stages in a woman's life when soy has vastly different effects. If natural estrogen levels are high, as with premenopausal women, soy isoflavones can block the negative effects of natural estrogens. For a perimenopausal woman, there is evidence that soy consumption can relieve hot flashes. However, after menopause, women produce very little estrogen, and in this state, high soy intake can have an adverse estrogen-like effect.[29]

I have this note of caution: There are people who do not tolerate soy. My clinical experience has it in the top five food allergens. I have seen several cases of allergic reactions from daily consumption of soy. Sensitivities to soy can be more difficult to detect because the symptoms can be subtle. Because soy isolates can be added to many processed foods, this sensitivity is easily missed. For those who can tolerate soy, I recommend it in moderation and only in fermented form (to avoid the mineral-blocking properties in unfermented soy). As mentioned in Chapter 1, much of the soy grown in North America is genetically modified, and the potential health risk of GMOs is another reason to avoid soy unless it is organically grown.

> When my son was a baby, we determined he could not tolerate cow's milk or formula made from cow's milk (a weakness he no doubt inherited from me). The only alternative at the time was soy-based formula, and because this was before my holistic nutrition training, he drank soy milk for a few years. I shudder to think how this may have compromised his health. Now in his twenties, he has some food and additive sensitivities. I wonder about the long-term health impact from his soy consumption at so young an age. At this writing, he is a young adult with no apparent ill effects, yet.

Grains as a Staple

Myth: We need to eat six to eight daily servings of whole grains for good health.
Fact: Grains have been modified (altered) to where, even in whole, unrefined form, they may be health hazards.

Two grains—wheat and corn—are the primary grain crops grown in North America. This is no accident. The federal governments in the United States and Canada subsidize cultivation of these grains. With all this home-grown grain around, is it any wonder that grains became a staple of our diet, and, that health authorities promote them? I suspect this led Canada's Food Guide (2011 version) to recommend a 35-year-old woman consume six to seven servings of whole grains per day.[30] As a nutritionist counselling in weight management, I know that this number of grain servings would fit the needs of a six-foot-tall man who exercises regularly. For the 35-year-old woman, six to seven grain servings do not leave caloric room for weight-modulating foods, such as vegetables, and would certainly promote weight gain.

In North America, most grain-based foods contain wheat, making it very difficult to avoid. As my clients rightly lament, "wheat is in everything." Not only is wheat in almost all breads and cereals, but it is also the grain of choice in cookies, crackers, pizzas, pastas, cakes, and pies. We all want these foods to be fluffy and hang together without crumbling and no other grain does this quite as well as wheat. A great thickening agent, it is also the basis of most gravies and sauces.

As revealed in Chapter 1, crop science has hybridized (altered) wheat to the point it does not resemble the wheat our parents and grandparents ate. Perhaps changes to wheat started with good intentions, to increase crop yields and hardiness. However, the unintended result was to increase wheat's gluten content, making it more difficult to digest and metabolize. Changes to wheat have made it a potential health hazard that has been associated with increased weight, joint inflammation, bone loss, increases in bad cholesterol, and accelerated aging.[31] Consider for a moment the health-care costs associated with the ailments linked with wheat consumption. In 2013, Health Canada listed wheat among the top ten food allergens.[32]

I maintain there are people who can still tolerate wheat but growing numbers of those who are intolerant, and not aware of it. Continuing to eat foods to which we are sensitive will cause health problems, eventually. I believe it is imperative for everyone to take a proactive approach and determine whether wheat is tolerated. In Chapter 8, I offer methods for identifying such sensitivities.

Because corn is a major crop in North America, and relatively inexpensive, it has found its way into many of our foods as a sweetener. Corn sugar, when processed, becomes high-fructose corn syrup (HFCS). A very common sweetener in processed foods, we often find it in cereals, cookies, soft drinks, fruit-flavoured drinks, yogurt, ice cream, and canned fruit. As discussed in Chapter 2, there are mounting concerns about the adverse health effects of HFCS. Corn is number three in the most common sensitivities among my clients (dairy is number one, and wheat, number two). Even without a sensitivity to corn, it can be difficult to digest and cause irritation in the intestinal tract. I routinely find that elimination of corn from the diet eases digestive distress among my clients.

In this chapter, I identify six food myths that could make a critical difference to health. Our ability to be well could hinge on avoidance of some of these foods. Having said this, we always fare better by acting on information that is personally relevant. If you feel well consuming dairy products, soy, eggs, wheat, and corn, then you may continue to have them in moderate amounts. If you do not feel well, it is critical that you determine whether these foods are healthy for you. I present methods of determining your tolerance for various foods in Chapter 8: Find Your Right Diet. Trans fats and damaged fats are not health promoting for anyone; their elimination is essential to being well.

Chapter Notes

1. "Lactose Intolerance: New Understandings" *National Dairy Council,* 81 no. 4 (July/August 2010), accessed September 12, 2014, http://www.nationaldairycouncil.org.

2. Yuval Itan, et al., "The Origins of Lactase Persistence in Europe," *PLoS Computational Biology* (August 2009), accessed June 15, 2014, doi: 10.1371/journal.pcbi.1000491.

3. Annemarie Colbin, *Food and Healing,* Tenth anniversary edition (New York, New York: Ballantyne Books, 1996), 150-1.

4. Mary Enig, PhD, "Homogenization & Heart Disease," *Weston A, Price Foundation, westonaprice.org,* accessed June 20, 2014, http://www.westonaprice.org/health-topics/milk-homogenization-heart-disease/.

5. Neal D. Barnard, MD, and Bryanna Grogan, *Dr. Neal Barnard's Program for Reversing Diabetes: The Scientifically Proven System for Reversing Diabetes without Drugs* (New York, New York: Rodale Books, 2007).

6. Amy Joy Lanou, Susan E. Berkow, PhD and ND Barnard, MD, "Calcium, dairy products, and bone health in children and young adults: A re-evaluation of the evidence," *Pediatrics* 115 no.3 (2005): 736-743, accessed December 5, 2014, doi: 10.1542/peds.2004-0548.

7. D. Feskanich, W.C. Willett and G.A. Colditz, "Calcium, vitamin D, milk consumption, and hip fractures: a prospective study among postmenopausal women," *American Journal of Clinical Nutrition* 77 (2003): 504–511, accessed June 21, 2014, http://www.ncbi.nlm.nih.gov/pubmed/12540414.

8. "Report of a Joint WHO/FAO Expert Consultation, Diet, Nutrition, and the Prevention of Chronic Diseases," *World Health Organization Technical Report Series* 916, (2003): 129-131, accessed November 17, 2014, http://whqlibdoc.who.int/trs/who_trs_916.pdf.

9. Sally Fallon with Mary G. Enig, PhD, *Nourishing Traditions,* Revised 2nd edition (Washington, DC: New Trends Publishing Inc., 2001), 15.

10. Frank B. Hu et al., "Types of Dietary Fat and Risk of Coronary Heart Disease: A Critical Review," *Journal of the American College of Nutrition* 20 no.1 (2001): 42, accessed June 15, 2014, http://www.ncbi.nlm.nih.gov/pubmed/11293467.

11. Sally Fallon with Mary G. Enig, PhD, *Nourishing Traditions,* 15.

12. Larry McCleary, *Feed Your Brain, Lose Your Belly: A Brain Surgeon Reveals the Weight-Loss Secrets of the Brain-Belly Connection* (Austin, Texas: Greenleaf Book Group, 2011).

13. Udo Erasmus, *Fats That Heal, Fats That Kill: The Complete Guide to Fats, Oils, Cholesterol and Human Health* (Burnaby, British Columbia: Alive Books, 1986).

14. "Eliminating Trans Fat," *Heart and Stroke Foundation, heartandstroke.com,* (June 2010), accessed June 20, 2014,

http://www.heartandstroke.com/site/c.ikIQLcMWJtE/b.3479251/k.5271/Eliminating
_trans_fat.htm.

15. Udo Erasmus, *Fats That Heal, Fats That Kill.*

16. Sally Fallon with Mary Enig, PhD, *Nourishing Traditions,* 14.

17. Dr. Ross Walker, *Highway to Health: Antioxidants and You* (Cape Town, Republic of South Africa: Dream House Wolcott), 42.

18. Frank B. Hu, et al., "Types of Dietary Fat and Risk of Coronary Heart Disease: A Critical Review."

19. Robert H. Lustig, MD, MSL, *Fat Chance: Beating the Odds against Sugar, Processed Foods, Obesity and Disease* (New York, New York: Hudson Street Press, Penguin Group, 2013), 110.

20. Sally Fallon with Mary G. Enig, PhD, *Nourishing Traditions,* 8.

21. Fred A. Kummerow, "Interaction between sphingomyelin and oxysterols contributes to atherosclerosis and sudden death," *American Journal of Cardiovascular Disease* 3 no.1 (2013): 17-26, accessed September 10, 2014, http://www.ncbi.nlm.nih.gov/pmc/articles/PMC3584645/.

22. Amit Sachdeva, et al., "Lipid levels in patients hospitalized with coronary artery disease: An analysis of 136,905 hospitalizations in 'Get with the Guidelines,'" *American Heart Journal* 157 no.1 (2009):111-117, accessed September 11, 2014, doi: http://dx.doi.org/10.1016/j.ahj.2008.08.010.

23. Dr. Dean Ornish, MD, *Dr. Dean Ornish's Program for Reversing Heart Disease: The Only System Scientifically Proven to Reverse Heart Disease without Drugs or Surgery* (New York, New York: Ballantyne Books, 1990), 25.

24. "Eggs and Heart Disease," *Harvard School of Public Health, The Nutrition Source,* accessed August 12, 2014, www.hsph.harvard.edu/nutritionsource/eggs/.

25. Y. Zhou et al., "The Effect of Soy Food on Mineral Status in Premenopausal Women," *Journal of Women's Health* 20 no.5 (May 2011): 771-80, accessed August 12, 2014, http://www.ncbi.nlm.nih.gov/pubmed/21486162.

26. "Too Much Soy Could Lead to Kidney Stones," *American Chemical Society* (August 29, 2001), accessed August 12, 2014, www.sciencedaily.com/releases/2001/08/010829083130.htm.

27. Sally Fallon with Mary Enig, PhD, *Nourishing Traditions,* 62.

28. Joe Schwarcz, PhD, *An Apple A Day: The Myths, Misconceptions, and Truths About the Foods We Eat* (Toronto, Ontario: HarperCollins, 2007), 64.

29. Ibid., 62.

30. Canada, Health Canada, "Canada's Food Guide, 2011," last modified September 1, 2011, www.hc-sc.gc.ca/fn-an/food-guide-aliment/index-eng.php.

31. William Davis, MD, *Wheat Belly: Lose the Wheat, Lose the Weight, and Find Your Way Back to Health* (New York, New York: Rodale Books, 2011).

32. Canada, Health Canada, "Wheat–One of the ten priority food allergens," last modified December 4, 2012, http://www.hc-sc.gc.ca/fn-an/pubs/securit/2012-allergen_wheat-ble/index-eng.php.

5: TOXIC THREATS

The accumulation of toxins in the environment over the past 50 years has made our bodies an ever-expanding toxic waste dump. ~ Ann Louise Gittleman[1]

Physical environment has a dramatic impact on our health. In the third world, where there is poor sanitation and contaminated drinking water, people have lower health status than those living in more affluent parts of the world. Unfortunately, North Americans also face environmental threats. Some are naturally occurring, such as heavy metals and infectious agents, while many more are synthetic chemicals. Exposure to such toxins negatively affects health in ways we will not immediately notice, because the effects can develop slowly throughout our lives. Understanding the sources and extent of exposure to toxins can help minimize their negative impact on health.

The increase in exposure to synthetic chemicals and radiation is the most dramatic of the changes in our environment in the past 150 years. In this chapter, I discuss environmental threats from various sources. There is air pollution from industry and car exhaust; indoor air pollution is also becoming a concern. Not only does our food supply expose us to harmful chemicals (see Chapter 2), there are also threats from household cleaners, personal care products, and the workplace. In his book *Never Be Sick Again: Health Is a Choice, Learn How to Choose It*, Raymond Francis states: "There are more than one hundred thousand chemicals now in commercial use, at least 25 percent of which are known to be hazardous; many others have never been tested at all!"[2] Low-level radiation has been around for millennia, but with the discovery of atomic energy and devices such as X-rays, televisions, and cell phones, we have dramatically increased our exposure. I also identify the health risks from naturally occurring environmental threats from viruses, bacteria, mold/fungi, and parasites.

Throughout a lifetime, it is almost impossible to avoid environmental toxins and their adverse health effects. Several reputable scientists, doctors, and nutritionists have warned how detrimental toxic exposure can be to our health. There is evidence of the involvement of toxins in the development of health issues such as behavioural disorders, learning disabilities, birth defects, and cancer.

Are We Toxic?

Two key factors determine our personal health risks from toxins: the extent of both exposure and absorption. To investigate the issue of toxin absorption, Environmental Defence Canada tested some Canadians for toxic residue in their bodies. Its groundbreaking 2005 report revealed that toxic chemicals (e.g., DDT,

PCBs, stain repellants, flame retardants), and heavy metals (e.g., mercury and lead) are contaminating Canadians. The report also revealed that these toxins contaminate people, no matter where they live, how old they are, or what they do for a living. The report outlines the risk of such contamination: "Canadian companies release many of the chemicals for which the study tested. Scientific research links exposure to toxic chemicals to many ailments that have been increasing in Canadians in recent decades, including several forms of cancer, reproductive disorders, birth defects, asthma and neurodevelopmental disorders."[3]

The Environmental Defence Canada study involved only eleven people. To be reliable, a study should involve a much larger group. However, there is still cause for concern because the volunteer participants in this study had a minimum of 32 of 88 toxins show up in the tests, even though they did not smoke; many ate organic food, and most led a low-chemical life. The First Nations participant had the highest levels of mercury, PCBs, and pesticides. Authorities in North America banned PCBs in 1979, but because they do not break down easily in the soil, the risk of exposure continues. In this study, even those born in the 1980s tested positively for PCBs.

In this chapter, I address toxic threats in four categories:

Heavy metals
Chemicals
Radiation
Natural infectious agents (viruses, bacteria, mold/fungi, parasites)

Heavy Metals

Even though heavy metals are naturally occurring in our environment, they are perhaps the greatest threat to our health. It is only in the past 200 years that we have come into contact with heavy metals in ways never intended by nature. Exposure began with the Industrial Revolution and escalated with the introduction of modern conveniences and products. Henry Schroeder, a former professor of medicine at Dartmouth Medical School, points to five toxic trace metals—antimony, beryllium, cadmium, lead, and mercury—that he believes are involved in at least half the deaths and much of the disabling disease in the United States.[4] Noted nutritionist Ann Louise Gittleman adds aluminum and arsenic to this list. These heavy metals suppress the immune system, accelerate the aging process, and increase the risk of degenerative diseases.[5]

Mercury, aluminum, and lead can be toxic no matter how minute the exposure. There is no test to determine how much heavy metal exposure we can endure because of individual differences or *biochemical individuality,* a central premise of the Holistic Model of Wellness. Repeated exposure and gradual accumulation in the body means we may not feel the effects for years. Talk about a silent killer! Much like taking out life insurance, it makes sense to avoid exposure to heavy metals. I offer the following guide so you can avoid the heavy metals that pose the greatest threat to health.

Heavy Metals: Health Risks and Sources

In this section, I summarize the health threats from five heavy metals, which, based on my research of the work of health writers,[6] government agencies,[7] and medical authorities,[8] I believe to be of most concern today—aluminum, antimony, cadmium, lead, and mercury.

Aluminum

Health risks: Ulcers, heart disease, memory loss, mental confusion, osteoporosis, Parkinson's disease, amyotrophic lateral sclerosis, impaired motor coordination, and Alzheimer's disease. Research has determined that aluminum exposure is a major risk factor in the development of dementia, in particular Alzheimer's.[9]

Sources: Antacids, pain relievers, antiperspirants, pickles, cosmetics, pots and pans (including "non-stick"), aluminum foil, canned food, and municipal water supplies

Most at risk: Almost everyone in North America, but in particular metalworkers, jewellers, and potters

Antimony

Health risks: Lung cancer, miscarriage, premature birth, disruption of menstrual cycle

Sources: Dental materials, dyes, pigments, lacquers, glazes, enamels, pottery, glass, abrasives, flame-producing substances, drugs for tropical diseases, ant poison, explosives, fireworks, and matches

Most at risk: Glassblowers, potters, painters, dyers, and solderers

Cadmium

Health risks: Cancer (lung, prostate), chromosome damage, bone pain, kidney damage, and reduced birth weight

Sources: Cigarette smoke or second-hand smoke; metal containers of food or drink; cookware with cadmium-containing glaze; pesticides; antiseptics; medications for dandruff and oily skin

Most at risk: Smokers, jewellers, potters, welders, painters, sculptors, artists, photographers

Lead

Health risks in children: Learning disabilities, attention deficit disorder, and hyperactivity. Environment Canada lists lead as a toxic substance. The Centers for Disease Control (CDC) in the United States calls lead poisoning the most common and socially devastating environmental disease of young children. In 2013, the CDC estimated one-half million children under age six have blood lead levels high enough to require public health action.[10] It is interesting to note that the CDC has not established a safe blood lead level for children.

General health risks: Vision damage, hearing loss, menstrual difficulties, kidney disease, miscarriage, convulsions, coma, and death

Sources: Older water pipes, paint (over 40 years old), window blinds, pesticides, cigarettes, cookware, pottery, old china dishes, canned food (imported), cosmetics (lipstick, eyeliner), and toys (imported)

Most at risk: Because of widespread exposure, almost everyone in North America

Mercury

Health risks: Damage to brain, nervous system, and kidneys, which can underlie several ailments such as depression, mental disturbances, high blood pressure, birth defects, multiple sclerosis. Sufficient exposure can cause death

Sources: Fish (bottom feeding, larger species, e.g., tuna), dental fillings (silver amalgams), mercury thermometers, pesticides, fungicides, cosmetics, waste incineration, coal combustion, base metal smelting, and the chlor-alkali industry, which produces chlorine, one of the most common chemicals used by industry in North America

Most at risk: Almost everyone in North America, but in particular painters, potters, metalworkers, jewellers, and anyone with silver amalgam fillings

Of the five heavy metals, aluminum, lead and mercury are the most difficult to avoid because of their widespread use in manufacturing and contamination of the food supply. The potential for toxicity is high. Assessing for toxic overload and the process of detoxifying the body of heavy metals is the focus of Chapter 15.

Chemicals

We are exposed to thousands of chemicals via air, water, food, and physical contact. As already noted, few chemicals have been rigorously studied for their health effects. A joint project of several universities in the United States showed that when wildlife is exposed to high doses of chemicals, there is increased incidence of malformed reproductive organs and sex hormone imbalances at a critical stage of fetal development. Liver and kidney function will be compromised over time.[11] If wildlife is affected, so are we. Some chemicals may be difficult to avoid; if we cannot choose where we live or work, exposure may be inevitable. However, we can reduce our exposure through our food and product choices.

As revealed in Chapter 1, pesticides pose a significant health threat, and this includes DDT, even though it is no longer in use. DDT was banned in 1972, but the risk of exposure continues, as explained in this 2011 statement by the United States Environmental Protection Agency (EPA):

> We continue to find DDT in our environment. Other parts of the world continue to use DDT in agricultural practices and in disease-control programs. Therefore, atmospheric deposition is the current source of new DDT contamination in our Great Lakes. DDT can take more than 15 years to break down in our environment. Fish consumption advisories are in effect for DDT in many waterways, including the Great Lakes ecosystem.[12]

The CDC considers DDT a human carcinogen that can cause damage to the liver and the reproductive and nervous systems. A long-term study has linked DDT exposure to increased risk of breast cancer.[13]

Even the manufacturing process for DDT has had disastrous consequences. In 1990, the water supply in the town of Elmira, Ontario, was found to be contaminated with *N-nitrose dimethylamine* after years of improper waste disposal from production of the chemicals DDT, 2,4-D and 2,4,5-T (Agent Orange). At this writing, the wells in Elmira remain closed; drinking water must be piped in from a neighbouring community.[14]

Organotin compounds are chemicals composed of tin linked to hydrocarbons, used in industrial materials and various biocides and fungicides (e.g., stannous chloride, stannous sulfide, stannic oxide, tributyltin oxide). Organotin compounds can enter the environment in several ways: seawater, seafood, fruits, vegetables, and consumer goods such as toothpaste, antifungal paint, dyes, and perfumes. The CDC reports the following potential health risks: stomachache, anemia, liver problems, kidney problems, neurological problems, skin, and eye irritation.[15] The CDC has received reports of ill effects but mostly among chemical workers and chemists who worked with these compounds. However, adverse effects have also been reported from exposure to antifungal paint used in homes. The next section deals with the most common toxic risks in our homes.

Household Chemical Threats

Exposure to toxic chemicals in our homes can occur through air and physical contact. Chemicals that we breathe in unknowingly are of particular concern. While air quality in manufacturing facilities is a concern, our own homes could be even worse. For those of us living in a climate that requires central heating, homes are closed up for several months of the year. Poor ventilation, combined with chemical off-gassing from furniture, flooring, and carpet, means that we may breathe in one or more of: formaldehyde, toxic flame retardants (PBDEs), and stain-resistant PFC chemicals (*perfluorinated* compounds). Other chemicals come to us in various ways through air, water and products that are in widespread use.

Formaldehyde is a known human carcinogen. The National Cancer Institute reports that research studies suggest an association between formaldehyde exposure and several cancers, including nasopharyngeal cancer and leukemia.[16] Fumes can trigger headaches and asthma. Household exposure comes from pressed wood products, flooring, coating for fabrics and carpet, paints, and varnishes. Fumes can be released for at least five years after a product is manufactured. Formaldehyde may also be in antiseptics, medicines, cosmetics (e.g., nail polish), wrinkle-free clothing, food preservatives, and pesticides.

Toxic Flame Retardants contain *polybrominated diphenyl ethers* (PBDEs). A study in 2002 linked PBDEs to neurotoxic effects, developmental problems and changes in learning and memory. Testing found PBDEs in human blood, adipose tissue, and breast milk.[17] Though there are safer alternatives (such as natural fibers),

PBDEs are used to make fire-resistant furniture foam, carpet padding, back coatings for draperies and upholstery, plastics, computers, televisions, building materials, and electrical appliances. Studies of exposure in homes found relatively high concentrations of PBDE in house dust.[18]

Stain-Resistant Coating for upholstery, carpet, and clothing contains *perfluorinated compounds* (PFCs). These chemicals persist in the environment, accumulate in the food chain (fish and meat), and stay in the human body for years. Studies have linked PFCs to immune suppression in children[19] and increased risk of obesity.[20] The extent of risk from exposure is not clear in Health Canada's position on PFCs:

> "Due to their persistence and widespread use, PFCs have been detected at low concentrations in the environment, food, and in human blood in several different countries. Based on the information that is presently available, the low levels of PFCs that are present in some foods that are sold in Canada are well below levels that are anticipated to cause adverse health effects."[21]

While this position makes risk appear low, young children and those with health conditions should still avoid PFCs.

Bisphenol A (BPA) from plastic containers can be released into food. As discussed in Chapter 1, research in 2007 confirmed the adverse health effects of BPA, which led to its removal from most plastics. While the official position on BPA is that of low risk, Health Canada has "recommended that the general principle of ALARA (as low as reasonably achievable) be applied to continue efforts on limiting BPA exposure from food packaging applications to infants and newborns."[22] Microwave cooking in plastic containers can increase the potential release of harmful chemicals into food. Will we ever know what the practice of heating plastic baby bottles in the microwave has done to the health of infants?

Chlorine is added to municipal water to kill bacteria, but not without negative health effects. Drinking chlorinated water can reduce the beneficial bacteria in the colon that are essential to digestion and immunity. Chlorine can interact with organic matter (dead leaves, soil) to form new chemicals called chlorination by-products. The International Agency for Research on Cancer classifies some chlorination by-products as possible causes of cancer, in particular bladder and colorectal cancer.[23]

Fluoride continues to be added to some municipal water supplies, even though, according the advocacy group Fluoride Action Network, there is little evidence that fluoride in drinking water prevents tooth decay.[24] Other sources of fluoride include some pesticides, bottled teas, fluorinated pharmaceuticals, non-stick cookware, and even some vitamin supplements. Controversy surrounds fluoride, in particular stannous fluoride added to toothpaste. Holisticmed.com states that, if ingested, it is a slow poison with these potential health effects:

Slow damage to the bones;

Interferes with key enzymes for digestion and metabolism;

Contributes to arthritic-like symptoms;

Neurotoxic (can lower children's IQ);

Increases one's chances of getting cancer[25]

In 1997, the union representing employees of the EPA voted unanimously to oppose water fluoridation in California because many studies had identified these health risks. The primary benefit of fluoride appears to be through topical application, rather than ingestion via water.[26] In 2006, the EPA's position was to regulate the amount of fluoride, while taking no official position on its role in preventing tooth decay.[27] In contrast, Health Canada's 2011 position continued to support fluoridated water for this purpose.[28] At present, some municipalities in North America continue to add fluoride to municipal water supplies, despite questions about its health effects. Fluoridated water often has a much higher lead content. The health risks from lead are revealed in this chapter under Heavy Metals.

Sodium laurel (laureth) sulfate (SLS) is a harsh detergent added to cleaning products that foam.

Health risks: Eye damage, intestinal damage, breathing problems, skin rashes and cysts, baldness

Sources: Shampoos, body washes, face washes, toothpaste, skin creams, and engine degreasers

I have assessed that some people are sensitive to SLS. They benefit from switching to personal care products that are SLS-free.

Polyethylene Glycol (PEG) is used to dissolve oil and grease and as a thickener in many personal care products. The David Suzuki Foundation reveals that PEG is likely to be contaminated with *1, 4-dioxane*, a known carcinogen.[29] However, government regulatory bodies currently do not assign health risks to PEG.

Health risks: Strips the skin of its natural moisturizing factors; suspected cancer-causing agent

Sources: Antiperspirants, lipstick, fragrances, pharmaceuticals, supplements, and even baby shampoo

Isopropyl Alcohol is an antiseptic and a solvent, which is made from petroleum.

Health risks: Inhalation and skin contact are the most likely means of exposure. Inhalation may cause headaches, dizziness, and incoordination. The CDC states that excess exposure can cause loss of consciousness, and skin contact "can cause dermatitis."[30]

Sources: Hand and body lotions, hair colour rinses, fragrances, aftershave lotions, massage preparations, cosmetics, and many skin and hair products

You might well ask, if all these chemicals are such a health threat, why do regulating bodies allow them in household and consumer products? It all comes down to diligence in testing. Unfortunately, it is only after chemicals have been in use for a while that studies find them to be carcinogenic. Consider how long it took to realize that cigarettes increased cancer risk. BPA was in plastic bottles for years before its ill effects were discovered. It is reasonable to expect there will be similar discoveries about other chemicals in the future. In the meantime, the onus is on the individual to be aware of potential toxic threats and try to avoid them. I consider it good health insurance to limit exposure to environmental toxins, even if scientific evidence of their threats is not yet available.

Radiation

Every day we are unknowingly subjected to radiation from natural sources, often referred to as background radiation. We have all heard of the dangers of ultraviolet radiation; too much exposure increases the risk of skin cancer. This exposure we can control; other radiation sources are more difficult to avoid such as radon, a radioactive gas found in soil, rock, and water. Radon also collects in homes; the EPA links such exposure to lung cancer.[31] Might this explain why some non-smokers develop lung cancer? Health risks increase from excess radiation exposure, but it is not always clear how much is too much.

My primary concern is the radiation through medical testing devices—X-rays, mammograms, and computerized topography (CT scans)—which can deliver high doses that are potentially damaging. CT scans of the chest and abdomen are equivalent to between 100 and 200 X-rays. Repeated use of these tests increases the risk of impaired immunity and, according the American Cancer Society, "may increase cancer risk very slightly."[32] The EPA has calculated that for the average person, 40 percent of radiation exposure comes from medical tests such as CT scans.[33]

In the holistic health field, it is widely accepted that overexposure to radiation can suppress immunity and increase the likelihood of serious illness. I find it tragic that some medical tests involving radiation are routinely used for cancer screening in spite of growing awareness of their potentially damaging health effects. A 2012 study in the United Kingdom found that among women who carry the genetic marker for breast cancer (BRCA1 and BRCA2), mammograms increased breast cancer risk.[34] The group that would appear to benefit from mammograms may be put at more risk. Mammograms are still the primary test used for breast cancer screening in North America.

Some threats from radiation are more difficult to avoid. People in urban centers are inundated with electromagnetic radiation, often referred to as radio frequencies (RF). Sources include radio, TV, cell phones, and wireless Internet. Studies show that risk is highest among those who work near TV, FM, and cellular communication towers. A recent meta-analysis of the effects of RF reported that the health risks of using cell phones were inconclusive. The fact remains that ill effects were found in *some* studies.[35] Unfortunately, the research to date has assessed health risks based on proximity to RFs over time, rather than on actual exposure. In the future, individual monitoring of RF exposure may give more reliable risk assessments.

Meanwhile, there is increased exposure to RFs in particular among those who use cell phones. Advances in cellular technology come at lightning speed. Most people are not aware that each new generation of cell phones increases the frequency of the electromagnetic radiation (e.g., 2G emits up to 900 MHz; 3G doubles the dose at 1900 to 2200 MHz). Research on the impact of higher frequencies (we will no doubt have in future cellular technology) has yet to identify ill effects. However, most studies, such as the one conducted by the Australian Centre for Radiofrequency Bioeffects Research, do not look at the effects of long-term exposure.[36] Because high-frequency cell phones are a relatively new technology, few people have been exposed long enough to evaluate the health risks.

Wireless Internet is rapidly becoming more and more available in businesses, hotels, cafes, airports, university campuses, and, increasingly, homes. Frequencies of wireless local area networks (LANs) can be as high as 5.7 GHz, which is an extremely high and potentially damaging frequency. Other short-range wireless devices include cell phone headsets and wireless computer keyboards and mice.

We now know there are energetic effects from RFs that *may* affect our health. Based on my clinical observations, RF's affect some people profoundly while others experience no ill effects. This is another example of how individual differences play a role in health risks. There is no way to know what cumulative effects from long-term exposure are doing to our bodies. For myself, I drive a car with a satellite antenna on the roof and a Bluetooth built into the car. At home, I have a wireless LAN, and I use a cell phone regularly. I, like everyone else, must consider the potential risk from RF exposure and either give up these technologies or reduce their effects by maintaining a quality diet and other immune-supportive activities (see Part 2 and Part 3).

Natural Infectious Agents: Viruses, Bacteria, Mold/Fungi, Parasites

Infectious agents have been affecting humans for millennia. In the 21st century, perhaps we feel less threatened by them because we have vaccines for most killer viruses. Water treatment has reduced exposure to bacteria and parasites. However, the evidence suggests that we continue to be exposed to infectious agents that have serious health effects. Few people realize that once we contracted viruses and bacteria, they can linger in the body as chronic infections, and cause ongoing health problems. A 2009 article in the *British Journal of Medical Practitioners* states:

> "Chronically ill patients with neurodegenerative, neurobehavioral and psychiatric diseases commonly have systemic and central nervous system bacterial and viral infections...the data suggest that chronic bacterial and/or viral infections are common features of progressive chronic disease."[37]

To this warning, I would add two other infectious agents: mold/fungi and parasites. Mold and fungi, normally present in the intestinal tract, can become overgrown and negatively affect health in several ways. I have observed that many medical doctors in North America consider parasites to be a tropical issue; their opinion could be responsible for missed diagnoses of parasitic infections, as was my daughter's experience.

To complicate matters, there is the controversial issue of vaccines developed to address several viruses and bacteria. In this section, I discuss the most common infectious agents, their health effects, and the holistic health perspective on their respective vaccines. This is not an exhaustive list of infectious agents, but addresses the most common concerns in North America.

Viruses and Vaccines

Viruses cover a wide range of diseases, some more serious than others. The virus that people are most concerned with is influenza, and epidemics are widely feared, most likely because of the 675,000 deaths from Spanish Influenza following the First World War. Since then flu outbreaks have not been associated with as much loss of life, and several predicted flu pandemics—swine flu in 1976, avian flu of 1997-1999, and, more recently, H1N1—did not happen.[38] Still, some predict we will see another epidemic on the scale of the Spanish Flu.

Each winter, medical authorities in North America advise us to be vaccinated as protection against the flu. Other viral diseases include rubella, chicken pox, polio, hepatitis, measles, mumps, viral meningitis, and smallpox. In the past 80 years, medical research has developed vaccines for all these diseases, the majority administered in the first two years of life. Vaccine Choice Canada makes this apt observation: "Since 1980, Canadian vaccine schedules have more than doubled the vaccines given; for the first 18 months of life alone, public health authorities across Canada now recommend 32-41 (average 36) doses of thirteen to sixteen different vaccines."[39] In recent years, new adult immunizations became available for shingles and the human papilloma virus.

Beyond the threat of viral epidemics, there are growing concerns that taking all these vaccines represents a dangerous assault on our health. The currently available vaccines often contain preservatives, the most common being *thimerosal*, which contains mercury—a heavy metal with many health risks—and formaldehyde. Canadian physician Zoltan Rona warns of other potentially harmful ingredients—monosodium glutamate and aluminum gels.[40] Although there is no proven link, the Vaccination Risk Awareness Network refers to the possible links between vaccines and the dramatic increase in asthma, allergies, attention deficit disorder, and autism.[41] The primary initial concern with vaccines is suppression of the immune system by preservatives and heavy metals.

I have personal concerns about adverse reactions to an anti-viral vaccine. In the preface of this book, I discuss my daughter's four-year bout of poor health after contracting an amoeba parasite—*blastocystis hominis*—but a vaccination may have been involved in its persistence. In the month prior to exposure to the parasite, she had received the hepatitis B vaccine—the first shot and the booster. My son was also exposed to the same parasite, but he recovered quickly. An obvious difference between them was that he had not received the vaccine. Of course, I did not connect these events until later. Apart from my daughter's reluctance to eat vegetables, the vaccine was the only other explanation for her immune system's inability to fight off a supposedly benign amoeba. However, no medical official recognized the involvement of the vaccine in her chronic parasitic infection. As a result, my daughter's reaction is not one of public record because there was no definitive proof that the vaccine was involved. This experience highlights the difficulty in assessing the risks and benefits of vaccines.

There is considerable debate about the need for vaccines between the medical community and the holistic health field. It depends on one's point of view about what determines health: is it all about external threats, such as viruses, or is it also about the terrain—the health and rigour of the individual? In my experience, it is both exposure to a virus and individual health status that determine the risk. When there is a virus going around, not everyone catches it; it is those with weakened immune systems who typically fall ill.

We cannot possibly vaccinate for every virus that exists. For example, Epstein Barr is one of the most common viruses, and the one that underlies mononucleosis. The information website E-medicine Health reports that Epstein Barr can also linger in the body as a latent infection and cause problems years after the initial infection. Because it is a living virus, it can become reactivated if the immune system is not working properly. A common latent effect of Epstein Barr is chronic fatigue syndrome, which is called a syndrome because its exact causes are unknown.[42]

Bacteria and Vaccines

It is important to realize that we live in a literal sea of bacteria, only some of which are harmful. Beneficial intestinal bacteria are essential for supporting digestion and protect the intestinal lining. However, there is also a host of harmful bacteria that, if too numerous, will cause illness. Streptococcus and staphylococcus are two commonly known bacteria that can cause either acute or chronic illness. Acute illness from a strep infection will manifest as an extremely sore throat, fever, fatigue, headache, and even gastrointestinal upset. Chronic bacterial infections depress the immune response, which increases the risk of illness. Before you run for the anti-bacterial hand sanitizer, be aware that bacterial infections can only take hold when immune systems are already suppressed or overloaded. For example, a viral infection can depress immune function and increase susceptibility to a bacterial infection, explaining why some people develop pneumonia after a prolonged viral infection.

Other bacterial infections can become chronic. *Helicobacter pylori* can proliferate in the stomach and, if undetected, can trigger stomach ulcers. Bacterial infections can also linger in the roots of teeth, and root canal procedures increase the risk. "Dental seepage" is the term used to describe bacteria leaking from the roots of teeth. There is growing acceptance that dental seepage from lingering bacterial infections aggravates cardiovascular health problems.

Vaccines exist for bacteria-based illnesses such as diphtheria, pertussis, tetanus, and bacterial meningitis. Like viral vaccines, there are ingredients with potential health risks. My personal experience with a common bacterial vaccine is not positive.

At four months of age, my son had pneumonia. Much later I realized this had happened directly after the DTP (diphtheria-tetanus-pertussis) vaccination that is standard for four-month-olds. A study published at that time in the journal *Pediatrics*, which I read years later, showed infants who received this vaccine had a dramatic increase in fever, diarrhea, and cough in the month following the DTP vaccine.[43] My son was a healthy 10-pound baby, was breastfed from birth, and my diet and health were also good. This means he had the best possible immune protection, yet his immune system could not withstand the DTP vaccine.

The quality of drinking water has long been an issue because of the threat of illness-causing bacteria. Waterborne illnesses, such as typhoid and cholera, were commonplace in the days before water purification. There are still instances of contamination of municipal water supplies, such as occurred in Walkerton, Ontario, in 2000. A dangerous strain of *Escherichia coli* (*E. coli*) from farm runoff contaminated the town's water supply. Seven people died and 2,300 became ill. Some have lingering health problems, such as high blood pressure, kidney damage, and cardiovascular disease.[44] One of my clients had lived in Walkerton at the time of the contamination. She fell ill but was not hospitalized. When she consulted me in 2014, she was still suffering from gastrointestinal problems.

Molds/Fungi

In addition to bacteria, the human intestinal tract naturally contains mold and fungi. It is not their existence that causes health issues; rather it is their overgrowth beyond a healthy balance that is problematic. A mold/fungi overgrowth causes poor function of the intestinal tract. Eventually, this will affect many body systems—hormones, skin, and nervous system—resulting in health issues such as skin rashes, athlete's foot, vaginal yeast infections, poor memory, anxiety, and irritability. If this imbalance continues, the immune system can be suppressed or become over-reactive—the latter scenario, according to nutritionist and author Jeanne Marie Martin, often results in autoimmune disease.[45]

There are a few ways that mold/fungi can become overgrown in the digestive tract. Mold/fungi can be ingested through foods: mold on foods such as cheese, fruits, and foods stored in the fridge too long. Repeated exposure to antibiotics favours the overgrowth of mold and fungi in the digestive tract. Antibiotics destroy all bacteria, both good and harmful, leaving the door wide open for opportunistic mold/fungi. Other sources of antibiotics include commercial meat and poultry. A diet too high in sugar will feed a mold/fungi imbalance. Because of the different ways it can affect the body, a mold/fungus overgrowth can be missed and go untreated. Identifying and addressing this condition is covered in Chapter 14.

Parasites

Health threats from parasites are more serious than most people realize. The National Institute of Allergy and Infectious Diseases reported in 1993 that parasites affected the health of millions of people in the United States.[46] Meanwhile, there are estimates that 85 percent of the North American population carries a parasite that impairs their body functions. The word "estimate" is used because parasites often go undetected. Parasites exist in a symbiotic relationship with us; they do not want to kill us, just feed off us. Their existence relies ongoing undetected. Meanwhile, medical tests for parasites can find only between 40 and 50 of the thousands of species that can infect the body.

It is important to distinguish between acute and chronic parasitic infections. Acute infections are easily detected because of the sudden onset and severity of symptoms. For some individuals, the parasite is never eliminated, and a chronic infection results. In 2004, a British study reported on 2072 former British servicemen who had been prisoners of war in the Far East during World War II. Years after the war, 12 percent were still infected with a parasite called *Strongyloides* that was common to the area of their imprisonment.[47] The CDC reveals that *Giardia lamblia* is one parasite of particular concern in North America for two reasons: it can survive chlorine disinfection in municipal water supplies and it can be transmitted person to person. The incidence in developed countries is estimated at 25 percent in adults and 8 percent in children. In developing countries, the infection rate is much higher at 33 percent. This means that international travel increases the risk of infection.[48] According to the CDC, one of the greatest parasitic hazards in the United States is a highly infectious species called *Cryptosporidium parvum*. This parasite can be contracted through the food supply, e.g., unwashed raw produce. Like Giardia, it can resist chlorine treatment.[49] This means that drinking tap water might expose us to *Cryptosporidium* and *Giardia*.

In my clinical practice, I have seen several people with symptoms of a parasitic infection that may have been present for years. They may not be severely ill, but their functioning has been adversely affected. Because there are numerous kinds of parasites with varying effects on the human body, several health problems and illnesses can result. My training, clinical experience, and research revealed:

- Parasites will reduce the ability to absorb nutrients and create nutritional deficiencies such as iron, B12, and zinc. Anemia (iron deficiency) is a common result.
- Parasites impair the intestinal lining, which can manifest as food intolerances and allergies.
- Due to the damage they cause to the intestinal tract, parasites are often involved in irritable bowel syndrome and bowel disease, such as Crohn's.

Research and the experience of holistic practitioners have connected parasites with several health conditions:

- A British study in 2013 implicated chronic Giardiasis in the development of chronic fatigue syndrome.[50]
- Naturopath Carolee Bateson-Koch has found that a tapeworm infection can underlie hypoglycemia (blood sugar imbalances).[51]
- Dr. Huldah Clark, renowned for research on the effects of parasites, reports that microscopic parasites can get into joints and eat the calcium linings of bones, leading to arthritis.[52]

In holistic nutrition practice, symptoms can be the best indicator of parasitic infections. Chapter 14 outlines the symptom patterns associated with parasites and natural healing protocols to address them.

It is critical to realize that some people never fully recover the health they enjoyed before becoming infected with bacteria, viruses, mold/fungi, and parasites. If these lingering infections are not detected and addressed, chronic health conditions can result, such as cardiovascular disease, irritable bowel disease, autoimmune disorders, arthritis, and osteoporosis. Whatever the diagnosis, a lingering infection could be involved.

Because of the prevalence in our environment of heavy metals, chemicals, radiation, and infectious agents, it makes sense to take precautions to limit exposure. This will pay huge health dividends, perhaps not today, but some time in your life. Choices (food, water, and products) that will limit your exposure to toxins are outlined in Chapter 7. If, after reading this chapter, you believe you have been overexposed to toxins, I urge you to refer to Chapter 14 and Chapter 15, in which I outline holistic nutrition protocols for cleansing and detoxification.

Chapter Notes

1. Ann Louise Gittleman, MS, CNS, *How to Stay Young and Healthy in a Toxic World* (Los Angeles, California: Keats Publishing, 1999), 2.

2. Raymond Francis, MSc, *Never Be Sick Again: Health Is a Choice, Learn How to Choose It* (Deerfield Beach, Florida: Health Communications, Inc., 2002), 149.

3. "Toxic Nation: Canadian Body Burden," *Environmental Defence Canada, Ewg.org* (November 9, 2005), accessed June 10, 2014, http://environmentaldefence.ca/reports/toxic-nation-report-pollution-canadians.

4. Henry A. Schroeder, MD, *The Poisons Around Us: The Unseen Dangers in Our Air, Water, Cookware and Food, and Their Leading Roles in Sickness and Death* (London, England: Keats Publishing, 1994).

5. Anne Louise Gittleman, *How to Stay Young and Healthy in a Toxic World*, 61-72.

6. Ibid; Danielle Perrault, RHN, *Nutritional Symptomatology* (Richmond Hill, Ontario: CSNN Publishing, a division of the Canadian School of Natural Nutrition, 2000), 116-8.

7. Canada, Environment Canada, "Pollution and Waste—Sources of Mercury," last modified July 9, 2013, http://ec.gc.ca/mercure-mercury/default.asp?lang=En&n=EB9F5205-1; United States, Centers for Disease Control and Prevention, "Agency for Toxic Substances and Disease Registry," last modified December 3, 2014, http://www.atsdr.cdc.gov/.

8. "Diseases and Conditions," *Mayo Clinic, mayoclinic.org,* accessed June 20, 2014, http://www.mayoclinic.org/diseases-conditions/.

9. Dr. Michael A.Weiner, *Reducing the Risk of Alzheimer's* (New York, New York: Stein & Day, 1987).

10. United States, Centers for Disease Control and Prevention, "Lead," last modified June 19, 2014, http://www.cdc.gov/nceh/lead/.

11. "Toxicology Information Briefs," *The EXtension TOXicology NETwork, University of California-Davis, Oregon State University, Michigan State University, Cornell University, and the University of Idaho, Extoxnet.orst.edu* (September 1993), accessed June 21, 2014, http://extoxnet.orst.edu/.

12. United States Environmental Protection Agency, "Persistent Bioaccumulative and Toxic (PBT) Chemical Program, *DDT,"* last modified April 18, 21011, http://www.epa.gov/pbt/pubs/ddt.htm.

13. B.A. Cohn et al., "DDT and Breast Cancer in Young Women: New Data on the Significance of Age at Exposure," *Environmental Health Perspectives* 115 (2007): 1406–1414, accessed June 20, 2014, http://www.ncbi.nlm.nih.gov/pubmed/17938728.

14. Bob Burtt, *No Guardians at the Gate: The Elmira Water Crisis* (Kitchener, Ontario: Bob Burtt, 2014).

15. United States, Centers for Disease Control and Prevention, Agency for Toxic Substances and Disease Registry, "Toxicological Profiles for Tin and Tin Compounds" (August 2005), accessed June 18, 2014, http://www.atsdr.cdc.gov/ToxProfiles/tp55.pdf.

16. United States, Department of Health and Human Services, National Cancer Institute at the National Institutes of Health, "Formaldehyde and Cancer Risk," last modified October 6, 2011, http://www.cancer.gov/cancertopics/factsheet/Risk/formaldehyde.

17. Prasada Rao S. Kodavanti and Ethel C. Derr-Yellin, "Differential Effects of Polybrominated Diphenyl Ethers and Polychlorinated Biphenyls on [³H]Arachidonic Acid Release in Rat Cerebellar Granule Neurons," *Toxicological Sciences* 68 no.2 (April 2002): 451-57, accessed December 5, 2014, doi: 10.1093/toxsci/68.2.451.

18. HM Stapleton et al., "Polybrominated diphenyl ethers in house dust and clothes dryer lint," *Environmental Science Technology* 39 no.4 (February 2005): 925-31, accessed December 5, 2014, http://www.ncbi.nlm.nih.gov/pubmed/15773463.

19. P. Grandjean et al., "Serum vaccine antibody concentrations in children exposed to perfluorinated compounds," *Journal of the American Medication Association* 307 no.4 (2012): 391-397, accessed June 18, 2014, http://www.ncbi.nlm.nih.gov/pubmed/22274686.

20. T.I. Halldorsson et al., "Prenatal exposure to perfluorooctanoate and risk of overweight at 20 years of age: A prospective cohort study," *Environmental Health Perspectives* 120 no.5 (2102): 668-673, accessed June 18, 2014, doi:10.1289/ehp.1104034.

21. Canada, Health Canada, "Perfluorinated Chemicals in Food," last modified, July 14, 2009, http://www.hc-sc.gc.ca/fn-an/securit/chem-chim/environ/pcf-cpa/index-eng.php.

22. Canada, Health Canada, "Health Risk Assessment from Bisphenol A from Food Packaging Applications" (August 18, 2008, archived), accessed June 18, 2014, http://www.hc-sc.gc.ca/fn-an/securit/packag-emball/bpa/bpa_hra-ers-eng.php.

23. "Chlorinated Water," *Canadian Cancer Society, Cancer.ca,* accessed June 18, 2014, http://www.cancer.ca/en/prevention-and-screening/be-aware/harmful-substances-and-environmental-risks/chlorinated-water/?region=on.

24. "Fluoride and Teeth," *Fluoride Action Network, Fluoridealert.org,* accessed July 6, 2014, http://fluoridealert.org/new-visitors/teeth/.

25. "Fluoridation/Fluoride: Toxic Chemicals in Your Water," *Holisticmed.com,* accessed July 6, 2014, http://www.holisticmed.com/fluoride/.

26. "EPA Scientists Take Stand against Fluoride," *Holisticmed.com,* accessed July 6, 2014, http://www.holisticmed.com/fluoride/epa.html.

27. United States, Environmental Protection Agency, National Academy of Sciences, "Fluoride in Drinking Water: A Scientific Review of EPA's Standards" (2006), accessed July 7, 2014, http://www.nap.edu/openbook.php?record_id=11571&page=R1.

28. Canada, Health Canada, "Health Canada Statement on Fluoride in Drinking Water," last modified June 23, 2011, archived, http://www.hc-sc.gc.ca/ahc-asc/media/ftr-ati/_2011/2011_82-eng.php.

29. "PEG Compounds and their Contaminants," *David Suzuki Foundation,Davidsuzuki.org,* accessed July 7, 2014, http://davidsuzuki.org/issues/health/science/toxics/chemicals-in-your-cosmetics---peg-compounds-and-their-contaminants/.

30. United States, Centers for Disease Control and Prevention, "Occupational Health Guideline for Isopropyl Alcohol" (September 1978), accessed July 7, 2014, http://www.cdc.gov/niosh/docs/81-123/pdfs/0359.pdf.

31. United States, Environmental Protection Agency, "Radon," last modified February 13, 2013, http://www.epa.gov/radiation/radionuclides/radon.html.

32. "General Questions and Comments on Radiation Risk," *American Cancer Society, Cancer.org* (September 8, 2013), accessed July 9, 2014, http://www.cancer.org/treatment/understandingyourdiagnosis/examsandtestdescriptions/imagingradiologytests/imaging-radiology-tests-rad-risk.

33. United States, Environmental Protection Agency, "Radiation Doses in Perspective," last modified September 24, 2013, http://www.epa.gov/radiation/understand/perspective.html.

34. A. Pijpe et al., "Exposure to diagnostic radiation and risk of breast cancer among carriers of BRCA1/2 mutations: retrospective cohort study (GENE-RAD-RISK)," *British Medical Journal* 345 (2012); e5660, accessed July 8, 2014, doi: http://dx.doi.org/10.1136/bmj.e5660.

35. "Exposure to High Frequency Fields, Biological Effects and Health Consequences (100 kHz -300 GHz): Review of the Scientific Evidence and Health Consequences, Munich: International Commission on Non-Ionizing Radiation Protection," *International*

Commission on Non-Ionizing Radiation Protection, (2009), accessed Jul 10, 2014, http://www.icnirp.org/en/publications/article/hf-review-2009.html.

36. R.J. Croft et al., "Do 2G and 3G Mobile Phone Exposures Affect Working Memory in Children, Adults and Elderly?" Australian Centre for Radiofrequency Bioeffects Research (ACRBR), accessed July 10, 2014, http://www.ursi.org/Proceedings/ProcGA08/papers/K02cp3.pdf.

37. Garth Nicholson, and Jörg Haier, "The Role Chronic Bacterial and Viral Infections in Neurodegenerative, Neurobehavioral, Psychiatric, Autoimmune and Fatiguing Illnesses," *British Journal of Medical Practitioners* 2 no.4 (2009): 20-28, accessed July 12, 2014, http://www.bjmp.org/content/role-chronic-bacterial-and-viral-infections-neurodegenerative-neurobehavioral-psychiatric-au.

38. United States, Department of Health & Human Services, "Pandemic Flu History," accessed July 12, 2014, www.flu.gov/pandemic/history.

39. "Vaccination: The Basics," *Vaccine Choice Canada, Vaccinechoicecanada.com* (June 2012), accessed July 12, 2014, http://vaccinechoicecanada.com/about-vaccines/vaccination-the-basics/

40. Zoltan Rona, MD, *Natural Alternatives to Vaccination* (Vancouver, British Columbia: Alive Books, 2000).

41. Ibid; "Vaccination: The Basics." *Vaccine Choice Canada.*

42. "Epstein-Barr Virus Infection," *Emedicinehealth.com,* (February 5, 2014), accessed July 12, 2014, http://www.emedicinehealth.com/epstein-barr_virus_infection/article_em.htm.

43. L.J. Baraff, et al., "Infants and children with convulsions and hypotonic-hyporesponsive episodes following diphtheria-tetanus-pertussis immunization: follow-up evaluation," *Pediatrics* 81 no.6 (1988): 789-94, accessed July 12, 2014, http://www.ncbi.nlm.nih.gov/pubmed/3259305.

44. "E-coli Infection Can Have Long Term Effects," *Ctvnews.ca* (October 12, 2012) accessed July 20, 2014, http://www.ctvnews.ca/health/health-headlines/e-coli-infection-can-have-long-term-effects-1.989587.

45. Jeanne Marie Martin, with Rona, Zoltan P., MD, *Complete Candida Yeast Guidebook: Everything You Need to Know About Prevention, Treatment & Diet,* Revised 2nd edition (Roseville, California: Prima Publishing, 2000).

46. Ann Louise Gittleman, CNS, "Parasites: Alive and Well in the United States," *annlouise.com* (December 31, 2011), accessed July 25, 2014, http://www.annlouise.com/articles/192.

47. G.V.Gill, et al., "Chronic Strongyloides Stercoralis Infection in Former British Far East Prisoners," *QJM: An International Journal of Medicine 97* no.12 (2004): 789-95, accessed July 25, 2014, doi: http://dx.doi.org/10.1093/qjmed/hch133.

48. United States, Centers for Disease Control and Prevention, "Parasites–Giardia: Epidemiology and Risk Factors," last modified July 13, 2012, http://www.cdc.gov/parasites/giardia/epi.html.

49. United States, Centers for Disease Control and Prevention, "Parasites–Cryptosporidium," last modified October 21, 2013, http://www.cdc.gov/parasites/crypto/.

50. Kristine Morch et al., "Chronic Fatigue Syndrome 5 Years after Giardiasis: Differential Diagnoses, Characteristics and Natural Course," *BMC Gastroenterology* 13 no.28 (February 12, 2013), accessed July 26, 2014, doi:10.1186/1471-230X-13-28.

51. Bateson-Koch, Carolee, DC, ND, *Allergies: Disease in Disguise* (Burnaby, British Columbia: Alive Books, 1994), 95.

52. Dr. Clark Information Center, *drclark.net,* accessed July 27, 2104, www.drclark.net.

6: EMOTIONS CAN MAKE US SICK

I would rather know what sort of person who has the disease than what sort of disease the person has. ~ Hippocrates

The outcome of tuberculosis had more to do with what went on in the patient's mind than what went on in the lungs. ~ Sir William Osler, MD, Canadian medical pioneer

Our mental and emotional health play a critical role in our physical health. If our social environment has not been supportive, our bodily health is likely to suffer, but not always. Some abused children become emotionally scarred adults who also suffer with emotionally based physical illnesses. Yet others with the same experiences rise above these challenges. What is the difference? It is not what happens to us; it is how we perceive the event. Perceptions are influenced by various factors: upbringing, innate personality, social environment, experiences, and the culture in which we live. This means that how we respond to what happens to us is highly individual; there are no neutral experiences. Positive emotional responses have great healing power; negative responses harm health. After Stephanie Matthews-Simonton's work with cancer patients in the early 1980s, [1] Dr. Bernie Siegel was the first medical doctor to document and write about *miraculous* healings from terminal cancer through health-supportive thoughts and emotions.[2] Unfortunately, emotions can be difficult to control to effect such healing. A key question is *how much of our emotional response to events is within our control?* There are different views in answer to this question.

Nature vs. Nurture

From my university studies of psychology and social work, I recall the nature-versus-nurture debate. Which is more important to our emotional state—inherited personality or our upbringing? On the one hand, we know that personality traits can be hereditary and may resist environmental influences. Comparisons of identical twins raised apart from birth discovered they displayed very similar personalities and behaviours. This provides some support for the influence of inherited personality traits.

On the other hand, nurturing is a critical factor in determining mental and emotional health, as well as physical health. While studying psychology, I learned of studies in which monkeys raised without a nurturing mother were emotionally unstable and unable to rear their own offspring. Lack of nurture negatively affects both mental/emotional balance and physical health in adulthood. Emotional instability has definite physiological effects, which are discussed in this chapter. Traumatic childhood events can also affect health indirectly. From early trauma, dysfunctional social skills may result, which can reduce employability and earning potential. As a result, there is less access to healthy food and safe housing—both essential to being well.

Society is full of people who, having suffered sexual or physical abuse, are left with severe emotional scars that negatively affect their lives. Some repeat the pattern of abuse by finding a partner who treats them the same way, while others can break this pattern. Somehow, the latter group can transcend the emotional impact of the abuse. Renowned self-help authors and speakers Wayne Dyer and Louise Hay both had troubled childhoods. Not only did they rise above their circumstances, but their stories have also made a difference to millions of others. Dyer was orphaned and lived in a series of foster homes, yet became one of the most successful inspirational authors and speakers. Hay's parents divorced when she was very young, and she suffered sexual abuse from a stepfather. She admitted that for many years her traumas ruled her life and led her to self-destructive behaviours and later a cancer diagnosis. Not only did she turn her life around, but she has also inspired others through her books and speaking.[3] Dyer and Hay both show us we have a choice in how we respond to negative experiences.

Emotions Have Energy

By now, you may wonder: *How is it that a feeling can be translated into physical health effects?* This question is the subject of much study. Dr. Valerie Hunt, a pioneer in research on bio-energy, provided the first truly scientific understanding of the relationship between energy field disturbances, disease, and emotional pathologies. In her 1996 book, *Infinite Mind: Science of the Human Vibrations of Consciousness,* she stated:

> As a result of my work, I can no longer consider the body as organic systems or tissues. The healthy body is a flowing, interactive, electrodynamic energy field. Motion is more natural to life than non-motion. Things that keep flowing are inherently good. What interferes with the flow will have detrimental effects.[4]

I find the best explanation of how emotions affect physical health from the work of David Hawkins, whose extensive research identified specific energy vibrations for each emotion. In his book, *Power Vs. Force: The Hidden Determinants of Human Behavior,* he explains how the emotional states of scorn, hate, craving, anxiety, regret, despair, blame, and humiliation all vibrate at a low energy level that is not health-giving. Emotional states with high, life-giving energy include affirmation, trust, optimism, forgiveness, understanding, reverence, serenity, and bliss.[5] Hawkins arrives at this profound conclusion about the power of high-energy emotions: "Love, compassion, and forgiveness, which may be mistakenly thought of as submissive by some, are, in fact, profoundly empowering. Revenge, judgmentalism, and condemnation, on the other hand, inevitably make you go weak."[6]

Deepak Chopra distinguishes healthy and unhealthy energy a little differently. He states, "Healthy energy is flowing, flexible, dynamic, balanced, soft, and associated with positive feelings. Unhealthy energy is stuck, frozen, rigid, brittle, hard, out of balance, and associated with negative emotions. Grief is a state of distorted energy that can last for years."[7] Mental health counsellors acknowledge how grief can have acute negative effects on physical health. I have heard of older adults who so grieved the death of their longtime spouse that they died shortly afterwards.

The effects of low-energy emotions depend somewhat on the strength of our body responses—how well we are—but some undesired effects are unavoidable. Our body systems are intricately connected, and when one system is impaired, other systems follow. Nervous and digestive systems are the first to be affected, but soon there is a snowball effect on other systems.

Why Running and Eating Don't Mix

The initial effect of emotions is on the nervous system, which has two branches with opposing effects on digestion:

- The sympathetic nervous system is activated with emotional stress and suppresses digestion.
- The parasympathetic nervous system is activated when we feel happy and relaxed and activates digestion.

The nervous system has an on/off switch—when one branch is activated, the other one is deactivated. This is an ancient survival mechanism to martial energies for the task at hand. Prehistoric humans experienced stress primarily from physical threats, such as an attack by wild animals or rival tribes. During a physical attack, the sympathetic nervous system became active in delivering extra blood to muscles and release hormones to sharpen the wits, all of which increased the chance of fighting or fleeing the attack. At the same time, the parasympathetic nervous system that governs digestion was turned off. This was by design; digestive energies were not needed while dealing with a life-threatening situation. This ingenious reassignment of energies no doubt helped the human species survive in a world full of larger and more powerful predators.

Today, the threat of attack is rare unless you live in the wilderness or a war-torn country. However, our bodies are still hard-wired to respond the same way to stress, even though most of our stress is emotional rather than physical. In fact, our bodies cannot tell the difference between a physical and emotional stressor. With continual emotional stress, as we see in modern society, the body's stress response is "turned on" all the time, which leaves digestion continually "turned off." In this situation, digestion is incomplete, resulting in symptoms such as acid reflux, constipation, diarrhea, or abdominal bloating. If these issues persist, the body does not absorb nutrients, and eventually this negatively affects other body functions: immunity, respiration, hormone balance, and circulation.

The other response to emotional stress is activation of the hormone, cortisol. This hormone helps the body store calories for what it perceives as a threat to survival. However, cortisol-induced storage of calories ends up in fat cells. As a result, chronically high cortisol levels are associated with weight gain, in particular around the abdomen. Cortisol levels should decrease at night to allow the body to sleep. Unrelenting cortisol is often the underlying cause of insomnia.

Does Melancholy Kill?

Humans have long believed that there are connections between health issues and specific emotions. In *Power vs. Force,* David Hawkins states, "The medieval concept of 'melancholy,' for instance, connected depression with impairment of the liver; in contemporary times, many physical disorders have been linked with stress."[8] Both research and clinical observation have found emotional links to several illnesses, in particular cancer and heart disease. In his book *Love, Medicine and Miracles: Lessons Learned about Self-Healing from a Surgeon's Experience with Exceptional Patients*, Dr. Bernie Siegel explains the emotions-cancer connection: "There is experimental evidence that 'passive emotions' such as grief, feelings of failure, and suppression of anger, produce over excretion of hormones that suppress the immune system."[9]

A study ending in 2004 involving thousands of heart attack patients in 52 countries found the presence of psychosocial stressors was associated with increased risk of heart attacks.[10]

Stress can lead to the excretion of nutrients, in particular minerals such as calcium, magnesium, potassium, and zinc. Such nutrient losses have implications for the rising incidence of osteoporosis. Marc David, author of *The Slow Down Diet: Eating for Pleasure, Energy, and Weight Loss,* explains: "America has one of the highest rates of calcium intake in the world and still has one of the highest rates of osteoporosis. The successful equation for bone density is not about getting more calcium. It's about excreting less."[11] With stress-related loss of potassium, salt levels can become too high—a condition that can lead to high blood pressure. Stress is also a factor in elevated bad cholesterol (LDL) and triglycerides—both risk factors for heart disease.

Chronic emotional stress is associated with multiple adverse effects, such as:
Allergies
Asthma
Cancer
Heart disease
High blood pressure and increased risk of cardiovascular disease
Impaired immunity; frequent colds or flu
Irritable bowel disease (e.g., Crohn's)
Irritable bowel syndrome
Obesity
Osteoporosis

Emotional Investments in Illness

An insidious emotion can develop among those who have a long-term or chronic illness. Because of all the attention and caring from others, people with the illness can inadvertently develop a fear of healing. Unknowingly, the illness can become part of the person's identity. The fear is that, without the illness, no one will care anymore. This belief is unconscious and, therefore, can be a difficult belief to change. Carolyn Myss calls this "*woundology*"—identification with illness that prolongs it.[12] I have observed this belief pattern with some of my clients who also had difficulty in healing.

Our emotional balance has a lot to do with how we age. How old we *feel* psychologically can profoundly influence our physiology. Deepak Chopra has written extensively about how perceptions and feelings affect the physical body. He states, "Expectations determine outcomes. If you expect your mental and physical capacity to diminish with age, it probably will."[13] For example, the feelings, *I am old, so I cannot do that anymore* or *I am old, so I will get sick* can set us up for more rapid physical and mental decline. The prevailing notion is that aging is out of our control, but how we feel about aging can make a difference in our experience of it.

It may be difficult for most people to accept that we can attract ill health through our emotional state. Louise Hay speaks to this in her book, *You Can Heal Your Life,* stating: "Whatever we believe comes true for us … Whatever we send out mentally or verbally will come back to us in like form."[14] A negative expectation about an illness can help bring about the very outcome we fear. This concept has been called the "law of attraction," stated simply as, "like attracts like." The law of attraction was conceived over 100 years ago as part of the New Thought Movement. In 1906, William W. Atkinson used the phrase in his book *Thought Vibration, or the Law of Attraction in the Thought World.* Over the years, several authors have elaborated on this theme: Norman Vincent Peale, *The Power of Positive Thinking*; Napoleon Hill, *Think and Grow Rich*; Louise Hay, *You Can Heal Your Life;* and Wayne Dyer, *The Power of Intention,* to name a few. The law of attraction is also the basis of the film and book *The Secret.*

Mahatma Gandhi reflects on the complexities of our emotional and physical health with this statement:

Your beliefs become your thoughts
Your thoughts become your words
Your words become your actions
Your actions become your habits
Your habits become your values
Your values become your destiny

In Chapter 9, I offer a method for assessing emotional balance and principles that support an emotional state for being well.

Chapter Notes

1. Stephanie Matthews-Simonton with Robert L. Shook, *The Healing Family: The Simonton Approach for Families Facing Illness* (New York, New York: Bantam Books, 1984).

2. Bernie S. Siegel, MD, *Love, Medicine and Miracles: Lessons Learned about Self-Healing from a Surgeon's Experience with Exceptional Patients* (New York, New York: Harper & Row, 1986).

3. *You Can Heal Your Life: the Movie,* DVD, Directed by Michael Gourgian (San Francisco, California: Lyceum Films, 2007).

4. Valerie V. Hunt, *Infinite Mind: Science of the Human Vibrations of Consciousness* (Malibu, California: Malibu Publishing, 1996).

5. David Hawkins, MD, PhD, *Power vs. Force: The Hidden Determinants of Human Behavior* (Carlsbad, California: Hay House Inc., 1995), 69.

6. Ibid., 140.

7. Deepak Chopra, MD, *Reinventing the Body, Resurrecting the Soul: How to Create a New You* (New York, New York: Harmony Books, 2009), 44.

8. David Hawkins, MD, PhD, *Power vs. Force,* 215.

9. Bernie S. Siegel, MD, *Love, Medicine and Miracles,* 68.

10. Annika Rosengren, MD et al., "Association of psychosocial risk factors with risk of acute myocardial infarction in 11 119 cases and 13 648 controls from 52 countries (the INTERHEART study): case-control study." *The Lancet* 364 no.9438 (September 2004): 953-962, accessed July 20, 2014, http://www.sciencedirect.com/science/article/pii/S0140673604170190.

11. Marc David, *The Slow Down Diet: Eating for Pleasure, Energy & Weight Loss* (Rochester, Vermont: Healing Arts Press, 2005), 29.

12. Carolyn Myss, PhD, *Why People Don't Heal and How They Can* (New York, New York: Three Rivers Press, 1997).

13. Deepak Chopra, MD and David Simon, MD, *Grow Younger, Live Longer* (New York, New York: Harmony Books. 2001), 19.

14. Louise Hay, *You Can Heal Your Life* (Carlsbad, California: Hay House, 1999), 51, 54.

PART 2: HOLISTIC GUIDES TO BEING WELL

In this part, I bring together all I know about promoting health from a holistic perspective. I base these guides to being well on the latest nutrition science, my holistic nutrition practice, and revelations from personal and family health challenges.

Knowing is not enough; we must apply. Willing is not enough; we must do. ~Johann Wolfgang von Goethe, 19th century German writer

7: Quality Food and Toxin-Free Living

Don't eat anything your great grandmother wouldn't recognize as food. ~ Michael Pollan, *Food Rules*

As outlined in Part 1, numerous factors threaten the nutritional value of food—growing methods, modified food, hybrid food, processing, transportation, and cooking. We also have misconceptions about the health of some foods because of politics, flaws in nutrition research, and food marketing. The following guide summarizes my best advice for a quality diet that will support physical health. If you are already experiencing health issues, you will also need to refer to Part 3 for the holistic nutrition approach to restoring health.

Vegetables, Fruits

Fruits and vegetables are powerhouses of nutrition that are a critical part of a quality diet. Nutritional science has established that they supply us with vital vitamins and minerals. Their health benefits derive from compounds called *phytochemicals*. These agents have a powerful, positive influence on health. From a review of over 200 studies, two Canadian oncologists make this conclusion: "In general, individuals consuming the least fruits and vegetables are approximately two times more likely to develop certain cancers than people who consume greater quantities of these foods."[1]

Here are my recommendations for maximum health benefits from vegetables and fruits.

To have:

- At least one orange and one green vegetable daily
- Organic produce—locally sourced is the next best option
- In northern areas in winter, frozen vegetables and fruits are more nutritious than imported
- Twice as many vegetables as fruits per day—fruits are high in fructose, a natural sugar, and therefore not a substitute for vegetables
- Whole fruit instead of fruit juices—to further avoid high fructose intake
- Dark-coloured fruits are generally higher in nutrients
- Cultured vegetables—pickled beets, cabbage (sauerkraut)—to provide prebiotic agents that aid digestion
- Bake, steam, or stir-fry in water; add healthy oil afterward

To avoid:
Genetically modified (GM) produce. Organic produce is not genetically modified.

Top Five Vegetables for Their Nutritional Benefits
Leafy greens—kale, collard greens
Cabbage family – broccoli, cauliflower, Brussels sprouts, red cabbage
Garlic, onions, leeks
Tomatoes
Orange vegetables—carrot, yellow peppers

Top Ten Fruits of Benefit to the Immune System[2]
Wild blueberries
Cranberry
Blackberry
Raspberry
Strawberry
Apple—Red Delicious
Cherry
Plum
Avocado
Pear
An average size adult thrives on daily servings of four vegetables and two fruits.

Animal Proteins: Meat, Fish, Poultry, Eggs

Animal proteins provide all the amino acids our bodies need on a daily basis to maintain our body tissues, from muscles to internal organs. The source and processing of animal proteins will affect their health benefits. The following guideline will ensure that you receive maximum value from consumption of animal proteins. These guidelines do not apply to vegetarians and vegans.

To have:
- Ideally organically raised, i.e., organic fed, livestock, or
  o Free-range eggs
  o Free-range poultry—chicken and turkey
  o Grass-fed, drug-free beef—no growth hormones or antibiotics
- Small, cold-water fish, e.g., salmon, mackerel, trout, sardines, anchovies
- Occasional: Lean pork

To avoid/limit:
- Bacon, smoked, and deli meats—to limit intake of nitrates and artificial flavours
- Large fish such as cod and tuna—higher on the fish food chain and more apt to contain contaminants such as mercury

- Shellfish—many are bottom feeders, which means their diets include waste products from other sea creatures. According to Fisheries and Oceans, Canada, mussels and scallops may contain toxins at levels high enough to put human health at risk.
  Preparation:
- Bake, ideally at low heat.
- Barbecue only on a pan or foil to avoid charring—a source of carcinogens.
- Properly cook meat ensures that parasites, if present, are killed off. Tip: Use a meat thermometer to achieve the appropriate temperature.

Grains

As a source of carbohydrates, grains provide a wide variety of vitamins, minerals, fibre, and even some protein. The primary health issue with grains is ensuring that sources are whole grain, i.e., not refined. The following are my guidelines for grain consumption.

To have:
- Organic, whole grains—brown rice, basmati rice, wild rice, oats, quinoa, teff, amaranth, kamut, rye, spelt
- If tolerated, wheat that is "stone ground whole grain" or sprouted ("Ezekiel")

To avoid:
- Refined grains—white wheat flour, white rice
- Corn—most of the corn grown in North America is genetically modified
- Overly processed grains—flaked cereals, crackers, commercial baked goods that are apt to have damaged fats, trans fats, refined sugar, artificial preservatives, colours, and flavours

There is some confusion about the number of grain servings that make up a healthy diet. The 2011 edition of Canada's Food Guide instructs adults to eat between six and eight servings of grains daily.[3] For most people, this intake level would leave little room for other important foods, such as vegetables and fruits, and could promote weight gain. A moderate intake of whole grains is health supportive for those who tolerate grains. Chapter 8 explains how to determine if you are tolerant of grains. The specific quantity required depends on body size and activity level.

Legumes

Even if you are not a vegetarian, I recommend including legumes in your diet to ensure adequate fibre and to reduce reliance on animal proteins. Livestock production requires more resources—land, feed crops, and transportation to market—that strain the planet's ability to feed the earth's population. I believe that eating more plant proteins, such as legumes, could, in the long run, do as much to resolve world hunger as donations to feed children in the third world. Eat organically grown legumes if possible.

The best tolerated legumes:

Cannellini bean, green bean/string bean, jicama, northern, snap bean, white bean[4]

The least well tolerated legumes:

Peanuts and soybeans—besides being a common allergen, peanuts have ill effects because of their tendency to mold. As explained in Chapter 4, once soy is fermented (soy sauce, miso, tempeh), it is often better tolerated. Unfortunately, most soy grown in North America is genetically modified.

Fats

A cultural fear of dietary fats exists because of flawed research linking their consumption to heart disease (see Chapter 3), and myths about fats that persist to this day (see Chapter 4). Considering that our brains are primarily fat tissue, why would fat be a dietary no-no? Dietary fats are essential for clear thinking, balanced emotions, and sound memory. Healthy fats are the building blocks of sex hormones, a support for the immune system, and a metabolism booster to help maintain a healthy body weight. There is no support for the common notion that eating fat will make us fat. The right kinds of fats are critical to the cardiovascular system. We can liken ourselves to automobiles which require motor oil to operate; we also need to oil our engine parts—heart, blood vessels, nerves—to keep them running.

Choosing the healthiest fats relies on understanding a few things about their nature. Fats are very sensitive to damage from heat and light, and once damaged, they can be harmful to health. For these reasons, fats are best eaten in their natural state, rather than extracted and served as oils. We also need to consume specific kinds of fat. Two fats our bodies cannot make but need for survival are aptly named "essential" fatty acids—omega-3 and omega-6. Omega-3 fats are anti-inflammatory, while omega-6s are pro-inflammatory. Both fats serve important purposes in body functioning. Temporary inflammation is part of the body's immune response. Unfortunately, because of overconsumption of vegetable oils such as corn and safflower, the Western diet is often too high in omega-6 and deficient in omega-3. Udo Erasmus explains how excess omega-6 promotes chronic inflammatory conditions such as high blood pressure, high cholesterol, and immune dysfunction.[5]

I offer guidelines to ensure sufficient levels of omega-3 essential fatty acids:

To have:

- Raw nuts, not roasted or salted—walnuts and almonds are the best sources
- Raw seeds–flax, hemp, and chia are the best sources
- Cold-water seafood and/or their oils, such as salmon, halibut, sardines, and anchovies

- Expeller pressed or cold pressed oils—extra virgin olive oil, avocado, grape seed, sesame, coconut, as tolerated

To avoid:

- Margarine—See Chapter 4
- Foods high in omega-6—sunflower oil and safflower oil
- Commercial salad dressing and cooking oils. Extraction of oils from their source typically damages the oil. Dressings may also contain preservatives
- High heat with oils that contain omega-3s, e.g., canola—heat destroys this beneficial fat. *Cooking tip:* Stir-fry food in water and add healthy oil at the end of cooking
- Frozen entrees, frozen pizza, crackers, cookies, fries, and potato chips—all sources of damaged fats or trans fats. Canadian regulations require processed foods to identify the trans fats content on Nutrition Facts labels but no amount of trans fats is safe
- "Low-fat" or "non-fat" products—they almost always contain sugar and artificial flavours

In general, fats should comprise at least 30 percent of our calories daily. Several online nutrition calculators identify, based on individual needs, how many fat servings make up this percentage. Intake needs vary with body size and activity level. A larger, more active person requires more fat servings than a small, inactive person.

Dairy

Some people can tolerate dairy products into adulthood, perhaps because these foods are part of their ancestral diet. Nevertheless, cow's milk may not provide milk's traditional benefits because of modern-day processing—homogenization and pasteurization. Chapter 4 discusses the health concerns related to dairy consumption. For these reasons, I do not recommend drinking milk, unless you can legally obtain raw milk. In Canada, it is illegal to purchase raw milk unless you own dairy cattle. One enterprising farmer in Ontario sell shares in his dairy farm, so that "shareholders" can legally buy the raw milk, but the legality of this has been questioned.[6] Some milk products resulting from a bacterial process (yogurt, kefir, cheese) are easier to tolerate and provide other benefits, such as probiotics. Depending on individual tolerances to cow's milk (see Chapter 8), I offer these recommendations for dairy foods.

To have:

- Plain organic yogurt or kefir
- Organic, hard cheeses made from raw cow's milk
- Organic butter, no colour added
- Goat's milk

- Raw cow's milk—not legal by commercial sale in Canada and most states in the United States
- Alternative "milks," such as almond, rice, coconut, and oat

To avoid:
- Pasteurized milk
- Soft cheeses, e.g., cream cheese
- Cheese with some mold on it—even though you cannot see them, the mold spores have spread through the entire block of cheese, so scraping off the mold is not enough

Fluids

Our bodies are 50-65 percent water and therefore require hydration regularly. Water is the ideal fluid, but it must be free of contaminants and contain minerals normally found in fresh water. Even though tap water in most areas of North America is safe for drinking, municipalities chlorinate water and, in some areas, add fluoride. Municipal water treatment does not remove all chemicals and toxins.

Drinking water should be free of chlorine, fluoride, volatile organic chemicals, and heavy metals. If you drink water from a well or a lake, I recommend treating it with ultraviolet light to kill bacteria and parasites.

These are my recommendations for the healthiest sources of drinking water in order of preference:

1. Spring water from glass or stainless-steel bottles: Look for sources that are regularly tested and have accessible toxicity results. Spring water is the ideal source because it contains naturally occurring, beneficial minerals.

2. Water filtered with a solid carbon filter (not granular carbon). Adding ultraviolet light treatment makes this source another number-one choice.

3. Spring water delivered/stored in hard plastic 5-gallon jugs.

4. Spring water stored in 1-gallon jugs. Try to avoid the flimsy jugs because plastic residue could leech into the water.

5. Boiled tap water. Microorganisms can be killed, but any chlorine and chemicals remain.

Some vendors now use filtered water in their products, so check food labels. It is impossible to avoid chlorinated and fluoridated water if you enjoy eating out. The best you can do is control your primary water source at home.

Reverse-osmosis (RO) filtered water is a popular filtration method that I do not recommend, except in certain circumstances. This filtering process removes all minerals, both harmful and beneficial. Regular use of RO water can promote the loss of beneficial minerals—sodium, potassium, and magnesium—deficiencies of which are related to irregular heartbeat and high blood pressure. Cooking foods in RO water can leach minerals out of the food, thereby lowering its nutrient value. Those who drink RO filtered water on a long-term basis need to take trace minerals in supplement form to avoid demineralization of the body. Nevertheless, RO water has a therapeutic use because it latches onto toxins and assists in their elimination. For this reason, RO should be consumed only during a detoxification protocol (see Chapter 15).

There is a common belief that we need eight glasses of water each day. This could be too much water if you are eating enough fruits and vegetables, which are also fluid sources. Which would you think has higher water content—fruits or vegetables? Surprising as it may seem, most vegetables are over 90 percent water, while fruits range between 81 and 90 percent. Vegetables with the highest water content include lettuce, celery, cucumber, radish, and zucchini. Fruits with the highest water content are melons, strawberries, and grapefruit.

Other fluids, such as herbal teas, hydrate the body and provide important health benefits. Some people tolerate caffeinated drinks—coffee, green tea, and black tea—which, if consumed in moderation, are health promoting. For more on caffeine's health benefits and issues, see Chapter 12. Alcohol is to be avoided, except for red wine because it contains polyphenols, natural substances that are formed during the fermentation process. Moderate consumption of red wine has a benefit to immunity. However, I recommend one four-ounce glass per day, and only if you are in relatively good health. With digestive problems, liver stress or weakened kidney function (see Chapter 11), alcohol is not advisable.

Seasonings

The main seasoning to avoid is table salt. It upsets the balance between sodium and potassium in the body, which is the reason it can increase blood pressure. Unrefined sea salt is a viable alternative because it contains trace minerals in a ratio and proportion that do not negatively affect blood pressure. Seasoning food is important to enhance the eating experience. Several seasonings have no ill effects. I recommend:

- Organic herbs, e.g., basil, oregano, thyme, sage
- Garlic, onions, and chives—add to cooking to reduce the need for salt; provides antibacterial, anti-viral benefits
- Unrefined sea salt in moderation—it contains approximately 80 minerals in trace amounts
- Black pepper—well tolerated with health benefits (antibacterial, antioxidant)

Sweeteners

Because sweeteners can create health challenges (see Chapter 2), it is advisable to limit their consumption. Avoid adding sugar to food or drinks. Processed foods are often laden with sugar or artificial sweeteners. It is critical to choose products that list sugar towards the bottom of the ingredient list, which means the sugar content is low. With limited consumption as a guide, I recommend two sweeteners:

- Unpasteurized, raw honey: Honey contains immune-stimulating properties that are enhanced if the honey comes from your local area. Unfortunately, the pasteurization of honey destroys its health benefits.
- Stevia: A non-caloric herb that has a neutral effect on blood sugar (ideal for diabetes and hypoglycemia).

I also assign an honourable mention to evaporated cane juice. It is not refined and therefore contains the full range of vitamins and minerals found in sugar cane. You will see this in many natural or organic foods; however, moderate consumption is still advisable.

Storage and Preparation

As explained in Chapter 1, the way we store and prepare food impacts its health benefits. Here are my recommendations to maximize the nutritional value of your food:

- Eat fresh food as much as possible;
- Avoid all prepared foods with additives (preservatives, artificial flavours, and colours);
- Store food in glass containers as much as possible to reduce exposure to chemicals and heavy metals;
- Avoid storing food for long periods in the refrigerator to avoid formation of mold. It is most apt to form on cheese and foods that are high in sugar or starch.

Cooking

Methods of cooking food will affect the nutrients that are available to the consumer. The following are cooking methods listed in order from the most to least favourable for retaining nutrients:

1. Slow cooking at low heat is ideal.
2. Steam vegetables so they are al dente, not limp.
3. Bake at less than 300 degrees F. Slow-cook meat at 200-250 F.
4. Boiling leaches nutrients from food into the water. Save the water for soup stock to salvage some of these nutrients.
5. Barbecuing meats or vegetables to the point of charring produces carcinogens (toxins). To prevent this, barbecue on a pan or in foil.

These three methods are not recommended because of their negative effects on health:

- Frying: Damages fats; browning of foods such as potatoes and meat creates carcinogens.
- Deep frying: Damages fats to the point they become rancid. Damaged fats are a major cause of illness, in particular of conditions such as cardiovascular disease, immune disorders, and hormone imbalances.

- Microwaving: Destroys up to 97 percent of antioxidants in vegetables, making them nutrient deficient. Reheating leftovers in the microwave will destroy all remaining nutrients.

Eating Patterns

Bodily needs for calories and nutrients throughout the day are not negotiable, and when and how we eat makes a difference to the benefit we receive from food. There is a saying that breakfast is the most important meal of the day, and this has nutritional truth behind it. In the morning, our digestive ability is at its peak; by 1:00 p.m., it starts to decline. This means that most of our food should be eaten between 7:00 a.m. and 1:00 p.m. Unfortunately, many people in our society skip breakfast, while others eat very little breakfast or lunch. As a result, more food is needed later in the day, when there is less digestive power to deal with it.

Irregular eating patterns have physical costs. Missing meals will slow down our metabolism, which can play a role in weight gain. The worst time to eat is within two hours of retiring to bed because the food consumed then will not digest properly. Calories taken late in the day will be stored instead of burned, which results in weight gain. Some late-night eaters do not sleep well because they are asking their bodies to digest at the wrong time. A common result is nausea the following morning because food sat in the stomach too long and did not digest properly. It is important to note that morning nausea is also a symptom of digestive imbalances (see Chapter 14).

Fatigue throughout the day is often associated with skipping meals. Not having breakfast is like putting the cart before the horse. Throughout the day, we must play catch-up, burning calories before we consume them. As a result, our energy levels are always lower and our performance, both physical and mental, will be sub-par. Not feeling hungry in the morning can be a symptom of sluggish metabolism, which should be assessed by a holistic practitioner.

Other eating habits can lead to serious health issues. In our fast-paced society, there is a disturbing trend towards grabbing a quick bite while still at our desk, or while driving our car. Some skip lunch altogether. It's like taking nourishment has become an inconvenience. This has also become a habit at home. At mealtime, our attention may be on TV, the radio, or text messages from friends. These are distractions to a healthy focus on the task at hand—consuming much needed nutrition. In *The Slow Down Diet,* Marc David explains how eating too fast with little attention to the meal results in less blood flow to digestive organs, reducing digestive ability, and even slowing the metabolism. David warns us these less-than-ideal eating habits could increase the risk of bowel disorders, lowered immunity, fatigue, and weight gain.[7]

Many diet books recommend eating in a relaxed manner to support healthy weight loss. (I define "healthy" weight loss at one to two pounds per week). I have heard from several people who went on vacation and ate heartily, not calorie-counting, yet they lost weight. This is contrary to the view that eating more food always promotes weight gain. It makes perfect sense when we accept that eating in a relaxed state supports healthy digestion and metabolism. This is borne out by comparisons across cultures. The French have historically eaten more fatty foods than people in North America, yet the French have less history of cardiovascular disease. The World Health Organization reports that the rate of adult obesity in France is much lower than in North America—17 percent vs. 23 percent in Canada and 34 percent in the United States.[8] The Mediterranean diet is widely considered as the reason for the lower rates of obesity and cardiovascular in France. There is another explanation for less heart disease among the French; It could be more about *how* they eat. Their tradition is to take lunch breaks, often two hours long, and they apparently take great pleasure in the eating experience, instead of the common North American attitude that meals are merely time lost from work or play.

Awareness of the impact of these habits is the first step to making health-promoting changes. In my clinical assessments, I have noted that those who eat fast, or eat on the run, are more apt to have digestive upsets. I recommend the following to promote complete digestion:

- Eat slowly—take at least 20 minutes to finish a meal.
- Chew food well—after you would normally stop chewing, continue for five more times.
- Focus on eating without undue distractions from TV, computer, or cell phone.
- Employ the lesson of the French—enjoy eating and do so without guilt.
- Adopt the philosophy of a weekly *fun food day*, when a favourite food can be enjoyed without guilt. Allowing occasional indulgences relieves the feeling of being denied something, which no one likes. My experience of counselling people during weight loss is that total denial of favourite foods usually results in cravings that derail all good intentions.
- Breathing is critical to good digestion. While eating, stop every few minutes and breathe deeply into the abdomen. This brings much-needed oxygen into the digestive process to ensure more complete digestion and metabolism of food.

Environment

A toxin-free environment involves more than foods and fluids. It also relies on the air we breathe, household cleaners, personal care products, and exposure to electronic devices. Here is my best advice for toxin-free living:

- Air purification in the home is beneficial. This is more important when there are new furniture and rugs that give off chemical fumes. Alternatively, have flooring and furniture made of real wood.
- Use personal care products that are free of sodium lauryl sulfate, polyethylene glycol, aluminum (i.e., antiperspirants), and perfumes.
- Clean with nontoxic cleaners—vinegar and water is the best choice. If something more toxic must be used, wear a mask and gloves.

- Use fluoride-free toothpaste.
- If you think electromagnetic fields affect you, limit your exposure to electronics, cell phones, and Wi-Fi.
- When travelling, avoid local water and food rinsed in local water. Eat only well-cooked foods and drink filtered water. This is one time that the salad bar may not be the best choice.

The extent to which environmental toxins and infectious agents affect each individual varies. Some people will be more susceptible to ill effects because of genetics, past illness, current health status, and nutritional choices. Assessing susceptibility and addressing it holistically is discussed in Part 3 of this book.

Exercise

Regular exercise benefits the entire body and its systems—the cardiovascular, skeletal, muscular, immune, nervous, and digestive. It is well known that exercise is essential to build muscles and keep our bones strong. Less well known is that exercise stimulates digestion of food and elimination of toxins. Deep breathing that accompanies exercise brings oxygen into digestive organs, thereby stimulating healthy function—digestion, nutrient absorption, and elimination. Release of toxins through the lungs is also enhanced. The Framingham Heart Study, a long-term population study, revealed that regular exercise increased life span between one and 3 ½ years.[9]

The ideal type of exercise will vary according to individual abilities and preferences. My basic recommendations are these:

- Daily exercise of at least 30 minutes in duration;
- Activity that elevates your heart rate to a level recommended for your age;
- Activity that you enjoy and are more likely to continue;
- Higher level activity but only if physical condition and health status allow.

When in doubt about the right type, duration, and intensity of exercise for your needs, I recommend consulting with someone trained in physiology and body movement.

Unfortunately, some people tell me they cannot afford the healthy choices that I recommend. It is unfortunate many in North America cannot afford enough food for their needs, much less worry about its quality. I understand because I worked for several years in welfare services and with volunteer groups advocating for food security. While we need to continue to work towards ensuring that everyone has enough to eat, those of us with financial resources can make choices that make a difference, often in unexpected ways. If more of us would avoid unhealthy foods and products that are toxic, these items could be forced off the shelves for the benefit of all consumers. We have already seen food companies respond to consumer concerns by reducing unhealthy elements such as trans fats, aspartame, and sugar. Choosing quality foods and limiting toxic exposure improves our health, reduces our need for medical care, and ultimately, the financial burden we place on society. A healthy population is also more productive, which is important for a strong economy. In this sense, committing to the goal of being well is not just personally beneficial, but socially responsible.

This chapter specifies what makes up a quality diet, healthy eating habits, how to avoid toxins, and how to exercise for being well. In the next chapter, I present an equally important step—ensuring that your diet is appropriate for your individual needs.

Chapter Notes

1. Richard Beliveau, PhD and Denis Gringras, PhD, *Foods that Fight Cancer: Preventing Cancer through Diet* (Toronto, Ontario: McClelland & Stewart, 2006), 24.

2. Ibid., 140.

3. Canada, Health Canada, "Canada's Food Guide, 2007," last modified November 18, 2012, http://www.hc-sc.gc.ca/fn-an/food-guide-aliment/order-commander/eating_well_bien_manger-eng.php.

4. Dr. Peter J. D'Adamo, *Eat Right for Your Type: The Individualized Diet Solution to Staying Healthy, Living Longer & Achieving Your Ideal Weight* (New York, New York: Berkeley Publishing Group, 2002).

5. Udo Erasmus, *Fats that Heal, Fats that Kill* (Burnaby, British Columbia: Alive Books, 1986).

6. "Top Court Refuses to Hear Farmer's Appeal," *The Star, Thestar.com* (August 14, 2014), accessed December 9, 2014, http://www.thestar.com/news/canada/2014/08/14/supreme_court_of_canada_wont_hear_appeal_from_ontario_raw_milk_farmer.html.

7. Marc David, *The Slow Down Diet: Eating for Pleasure, Energy & Weight Loss* (Rochester, Vermont: Healing Arts Press, 2005).

8. "Global Database on Body Mass Index, an Interactive Tool for Monitoring Nutrition Transition," *World Health Organization, who.int,* accessed March 10, 2014, http://apps.who.int/bmi/index.jsp.

9. Oscar Franco, MD, et al., "Effects of Physical Activity on Life Expectancy with Cardiovascular Disease," *JAMA Internal Medicine,* formerly *Archives of Internal Medicine* 165 (2005): 20, accessed March 10, 2014, http://www.ncbi.nlm.nih.gov/pubmed/16287764.

8: FIND *YOUR* RIGHT DIET

Each person is biochemically distinct ·and has unique nutritional needs. ~ Holistic nutrition principle, Canadian School of Natural Nutrition[1]

The foundation of good health is adopting the right diet for our individual needs. Unfortunately, some researchers and writers focus on finding "the one right diet for all." This compelling concept might sell books, but I consider the elusive search for one ideal diet to be *dietary myopia*—the view that everyone should adopt one group or one individual's dietary habits. There is no one-size-fits-all diet. Human history, variations in cultural diets, and research clearly show that humans survive on a variety of diets. Recent research into epigenetics has revealed that diet affects health in very specific ways. By eating the right diet for individual needs, we can suppress genetic markers for serious illnesses. The wrong diet can unfortunately turn on genes that promote illness. Finding the right diet *for you* is therefore critical to preventing illness and being well. This chapter explores how to use the latest information on nutrition to help you find the diet that best supports your health.

History of the Human Diet

The human diet has evolved over millennia. Early humans hunted and foraged for food and ate what they discovered was edible: game, nuts, berries, roots. Judging by our domination of the planet today, the human species must have thrived on this diet. Today, some diet theorists applaud the "caveman diet" or Paleo diet as being the ideal. But is it? Just because our distant ancestors thrived on what they could find in nature, does this mean we will, too? As we will discover, diet preferences have changed radically since then.

Once the skill of cultivation developed around ten thousand years ago, farming and animal husbandry replaced hunting and foraging as the primary food source. It was easier to raise an animal for consumption than it was to hunt for it. In various parts of the world, this agrarian lifestyle was dominant for thousands of years. Most people in agrarian societies were involved, as workers or estate owners, in crop cultivation and livestock production. Both my parents grew up on farms during the 1930s and '40s, and they survived the winter because of what they had harvested and stored from their crops and gardens. But, of my twenty-four cousins on either side, only one is farming today. Today, raising crops is a business in which fewer and fewer people are involved. Gardening has become more of a hobby than a necessity for survival. This has changed the source of food and often its quality. In two generations, dietary habits in North America have transformed to favour convenience at the expense of quality. I believe this dietary shift has health consequences because of some interesting aspects of the human diet—ancestral and regional variations.

Ancestral diets

Humans in different parts of the world have long survived on a variety of diets. Different climates offer very different food staples. Diets in Polar Regions are high in fish protein and fat, while tropical climates supply more fruit, vegetables, grains, and tropical oils. As a species, we are adaptable, having the ability to adapt to diverse climates, altitudes, and diets. After living in one region for a while, cultural dietary preferences develop that carry on through several generations. Those who thrive on the diet are more apt to reproduce, and their descendants will be more suited to the local diet, which becomes the ancestral diet for people of that region. An example of this is in Eastern Europe, where agriculture and grain crops originated. Food activist Michael Pollan believes the descendants of this area are more metabolically suited to eating diets high in breads and pastas.[2] In the United States, the National Institutes of Health has determined that intolerance to cow's milk is more common among people of African, Hispanic, Native American, and Asian descent.[3] Cow's milk is not part of their ancestral diet.

Today, human migration has increased dramatically, and, in their new country, immigrants often stray from their ancestral diet—the one best suited to their bodies. As a result, health issues can arise. My clients who were born in Europe or South America do not tolerate the North American varieties of wheat and corn. They develop health problems, such as irritable bowel or blood sugar imbalances.

> One such client had emigrated from Mexico 10 years prior. He had gained 60 pounds and his doctor diagnosed him as pre-diabetic. On my recommendation, he eliminated dairy and wheat from his diet. The results were dramatic. He lost weight easily, and no longer had symptoms of diabetes. Foods that he did not tolerate caused severe health problems that he reversed by returning to his ancestral diet.

Even if your family has not migrated, you may not be eating your ancestral diet. As discussed in Chapters 1 and 2, the North American diet has changed and not for the better. Foods are preserved and processed to endure long transportation and storage. Added salt, sugar, and flavours tempt our discerning palates, but make our diets different from our ancestors' fare. Michael Pollan refers to long-term population studies that link rapid diet changes with the dramatic increase in ailments such as type 2 diabetes, autoimmune disorders, asthma, and allergies.[4] My own agrarian roots are recent, and I wonder if my allergic tendencies could be related to a move away from my ancestral diet.

We Are All Different

Within a society or culture eating the same diet, some will do better than others. In the 1950s, Dr. Roger Williams identified the concept of "biochemical individuality" to explain variations in how we respond to food. As individuals, we naturally metabolize foods differently, during either digestion or absorption.[5] As already noted, many people have trouble digesting cow's milk because they lack the digestive enzyme—lactase. There are also variations in the ability to digest proteins, carbohydrates, and fats. In her clinical study of nutrition, biochemist Dr. Johanna Budwig was among the first to link poor fat metabolism with malfunction of the gallbladder, immune system, and digestion, as well as several diseases and conditions—heart disease, cancer, diabetes, and arthritis.[6] Impairment in digestion of proteins can lead to poor muscle development, poor-quality hair and nails, and premature aging. For some, the carbohydrates they consume readily turn to fat, while others burn off their carbs efficiently. Such variations in metabolism also explain why some people maintain a healthy weight more easily than others. Our individuality can be based on inherited tendencies, but can also develop through life because of illness, toxins, or eating a diet not suited to individual needs.

Theories about the Right Diet

There are various approaches to determining *your* right diet. After several years in clinical practice, I believe these theories may apply generally but not specifically to the individual. Therefore, they have benefit as general guidelines. I present them here because they teach us something about variations in the human response to diet.

Vegetarian vs. Omnivore

There is ongoing debate about which option is healthier—a vegetarian or an omnivore diet. The basic difference between these diets is that vegetarians rely on plant proteins, while omnivores eat animal proteins. Many nutritionists claim that vegetarian eating is healthier for everyone. However, this position ignores two truths about the human diet that I have just discussed—the importance of ancestral diets and biochemical individuality. Some people may have evolved to thrive on vegetarian diets, but not all. Consider the ancestral diet of the Inuit people of the Canadian north—high in protein and fat, and *no* grains, vegetables, or fruits. In tropical areas, the ancestral diet has less animal protein, but lots of vegetables and fruits. Yet people of both regions survived for thousands of years on what is, by today's standards, considered unbalanced diets: one too high in animal protein, and the other protein deficient.

The China Study, a recent population study, showed that a vegetarian diet was the healthiest. Comparisons of diet and health status in different communities in China determined vegetarians had better health and less cardiovascular disease than those eating animal proteins.[7] This appears to be definitive proof of the superiority of the vegetarian diet, but there are several other dietary issues involved. While it may be true that for the Chinese, a vegetarian diet is more healthful, it is not true for all cultures. The authors of the study admit that rapid changes away from an ancestral diet can lead to health problems.[8] If the meat-eating group changed from a vegetarian diet within one or two generations, they may have suffered ill effects because they had not yet adapted to meat eating. Interestingly, the study found that a moderate intake of healthy fats was also involved in good health outcomes. I wonder if this study was as much about the importance of quality fats as it was about the superiority of vegetarian diets. It is always questionable to focus on one aspect of diet and make definitive conclusions about effects on health.

Some make the claim that humans do not have the digestive system suited to meat eating. Meat eating (an omnivorous diet) requires a different digestive tract than a plant-based (vegetarian) diet requires. In the animal kingdom, plant eaters, such as cattle and horses, have long digestive tracts, while meat eaters, such as lions and tigers, have shorter ones. It turns out that the human digestive tract is not like that of either a meat eater or a plant eater; we are somewhere in between. This also fits with humans' historical ability to adapt to a variety of foods and diets.

There are different vegetarians, each with their own nutritional challenges. The lacto-ovo type allows products of animals such as milk and eggs. A lacto-vegetarian would include milk, but not eggs. Vegans exclude all animal proteins, including milk and eggs. Without meat, poultry, dairy, fish, and eggs in the vegan diet, there is insufficient vitamin B12. As a result, vegans are at risk of developing a B12 deficiency, which affects the availability of folic acid and iron. Anemia is a common result. B12 has a critical role in the digestion and absorption of food, and without it, there can result fatigue, depression, anxiety, headaches, and memory loss. Strict vegans are most at risk and are advised to supplement with B12.

The stricter the vegetarian diet is, the more risk there is of becoming deficient in protein. Our bodies need twenty amino acids (building blocks of protein), but can produce only eleven of them. To have sufficient protein, we must get the other nine amino acids, called "essential amino acids," from our diet. Animal foods are *complete* proteins because they contain all the essential amino acids. Vegetable proteins are almost all *incomplete* proteins because they are missing one or more of the essential amino acids. The only vegetable protein sources that are complete protein sources are chia seed, flaxseed and the seed/grain quinoa. However, their protein content is lower, which makes it difficult to consume enough of them to satisfy the body's needs. The protection against protein deficiency for vegans who eat no eggs or dairy products is to consume foods that, when combined, provide all the essential amino acids. Otherwise, the body will not have all the building blocks for protein production and, over time, a protein deficiency will develop. Symptoms of protein deficiency include general weakness; anemia; pallor; lightheadedness or dizziness; nausea; cataracts; muscle cramps; hair falling out; and difficulty building muscle.

At one time, nutritionists believed vegans must consume all the essential amino acids at the same meal, but it now appears that having them within the course of a day will ensure sufficient protein intake. Based on the work of Frances Moore Lappé, I have compiled foods that, when eaten during the same day, will ensure that all essential amino acids are present. In line with guidelines in Chapter 7 about quality food, healthy sources of soy are fermented (miso, tempeh, and natto). The following food combinations each provide all the essential amino acids, which are of critical importance for vegans:

Rice + legumes

Rice + sesame seeds/tahini

Grains (wheat/spelt/kamut) + legumes

Grains (wheat/spelt/kamut) + sesame seeds/tahini + miso

Cornmeal + legumes

Miso + rice + wheat/spelt/kamut

Miso + almonds + spelt/kamut + rice

Miso + almonds + tahini

Miso + sesame/tahini + wheat/spelt/kamut

Almonds + sunflower seeds

Nuts (almond, cashew, Brazil) + legumes

Seeds (sesame, sunflower) + legumes (chickpea), e.g., hummus

Given the risk of B12 deficiency and difficulty in obtaining enough protein, I question the claim that a strict vegetarian diet is ideal for everyone. It may be right for some people, especially if it is part of their ancestral diet. I have clients who thrive as vegetarians and vegans, while others who do not.

Ratio Tampering Diets

High fat, high protein, low fat, low carb, high carb—all have been promoted as *the* ideal diet for everyone. I call these "ratio tampering" diets because they all propose a skewed ratio of the three major food groups—proteins, carbohydrates, and fats. Most of these diets are not as health supportive as their proponents claim.

In the 1970s, the Atkins diet was *the* weight loss solution. This high fat, moderate-protein diet was an easy sell because many North Americans love their meat, bacon, and sausage. There is some biological truth to this diet. Fats and proteins keep us full longer, which means we are less likely to overeat. Prolonged high-fat/high-protein fare results in the burning of body fat for energy (which is desired for weight loss), but this also creates ketones that stress the liver and kidneys. For this reason, the Atkins diet is primarily useful in weight loss and not as a long-term plan. With the recommended 20 grams of carbohydrates per day, even Dr. Atkins admits this diet is not nutritionally balanced. He recommends nutritional supplements to make up for missing nutrients in the diet.[9] Proteins are also the most difficult food to digest, and those with weak digestion may have trouble with this diet. In addition, the original version encouraged consumption of bacon and sausage, neither of which is health supportive.

Another way to describe the Atkins diet is that it is low in carbohydrates, which would naturally mean that there is a higher ratio of fats and proteins. A two-year study in 2010 compared the impact of low-carbohydrate and low-fat diets on weight and risk of cardiovascular disease. The low-carbohydrate regimen had better results than the low-fat diet in relation to weight loss and reduction in cardiovascular disease risk factors.[10] The low-carbohydrate diet provided only around 20 grams of carbohydrates per day. To put this in perspective, adults typically consume from 150 to 200 grams in a day. It turns out this study involved only people considered obese. They could survive, for a time, on 20 grams of carbohydrates because they can use their own body fat for energy. Using body fat stores instead of carbohydrates for energy will trigger weight loss. There is another explanation for the reduced risk of cardiovascular disease from this diet—it could have as much to do with the weight loss the diet triggered than with the low carbohydrate intake.

I recommend temporary reductions in carbohydrates to help my clients lose weight. However, the daily intake of 20 grams of carbohydrate is extremely low. I do not recommend it for any length of time because carbohydrates are the primary source of energy for critical body functions.

In the 1980s, Nathan Pritikin promoted a low-fat diet to combat heart disease. He had found the low-fat approach addressed his own and others' cardiovascular issues. His heart disease was relieved, but sadly, he died of leukemia at age 69. This led to questions about the overall value of his low-fat diet. The Harvard School of Public Health has since reviewed all the studies on low-fat diets in relation to cardiovascular disease and reported:

> It is now increasingly recognized that the low-fat campaign has been based on little scientific evidence and may have caused unintended health consequences…. Only one study has ever found a positive association between saturated fat intake and risk of coronary heart disease, a weak and non-significant positive association.[11]

Some weight-loss programs continue to promote a low-fat diet. This may work for a while, but many of my clients who had previously tried low-fat diets reported they were too hungry to stick with the regimen. Because fats are essential for energy and cognitive ability, too little dietary fat leads to fatigue and foggy thinking. Fats are also essential building blocks for sex hormones; a low-fat diet can upset hormone balance (e.g., PMS, menopausal symptoms). I must stress that only the healthy fats recommended in Chapter 7 promote hormone balance.

The China Study, besides proposing vegetarian eating, concluded that eating less protein would make us healthier. The researchers observed that the health of its Chinese study group was better on low-protein diets.[12] Other research has linked low-protein diets with lower risk of cancer, however, in combination with other factors—healthy body weight and regular exercise.[13] All my experience in holistic nutrition practice has showed me it is highly questionable to claim that one nutrient is responsible for desired health outcomes. As my Holistic Model of Wellness outlines, nutrition, environment, movement, and individual responses work synergistically to support our health. Regarding ratio-tampering diets, they stray too far from the still-sound nutritional advice to "eat a balanced diet."

Typing Systems

In recent years, diet theories have emerged based on our individual characteristics and responses to food. These theories form a system for grouping us in *metabolic types* according to aspects of our ancestry and/or current relationship to food. The Metabolic Typing Diet[14] is one system that is also the basis for an online typing assessment promoted by Dr. Joseph Mercola.[15] I have not found these approaches particularly useful. Here I outline the typing system I have found most effective in helping my clients find their right diet. It all starts with typing based on blood, but it does not end there.

In the 1990s, naturopath Peter D'Adamo proposed that blood type—O, A, AB, and B—helps to determine the foods best suited to our needs. For each blood type, foods and beverages fall into three categories: beneficial, neutral, and "avoid." The four blood types represent human evolution, with type O being the oldest, followed by A, B, and, most recently, AB. Because the O blood type developed earliest, the theory is that today those with this blood type will thrive on the oldest diet, or "caveman" diet—wild game, nuts, seeds, vegetables, and few grains and dairy foods. Type A blood represents an adaptation to an agrarian lifestyle and is better suited to protein sources from livestock, such as chicken and turkey. Because type Bs developed later, they tolerate dairy products and eggs the best of all types. Type AB individuals are the most likely of all four types to thrive on vegetarian proteins.[16]

The blood type diet provides specific direction for all food groups—grains, vegetables, fruits, fats, herbs, spices, and even nutritional supplements. Some of my clients feel better following the blood type diet, while others do not. In my estimation, basing our diet choices on one factor—blood type—is too simplistic. There is no allowance in this system for what happens after birth, such as dietary choices, illness, and environmental influences. Peter D'Adamo no doubt realized these limitations and developed a new system called "genotyping." He based the system on "interactions between our genetic heritage, prenatal experience and our daily interaction with our environment, including diet and exercise. These elements and the way they interact fall into predictable patterns."[17] Calculation of the genotype diet considers multiple factors that represent our interaction with our environment since conception. The six genotypes are *Hunter, Gatherer, Teacher, Explorer, Warrior*, and *Nomad*. Each type relates to a different stage in the evolution of the human diet.

Genotyping is based on the recently discovered concept of epigenetics, which holds that diet and environment will determine how our genes express to either increase or decrease our risk of illness. A 2010 review of the research on epigenetics and nutrition made these conclusions: "During our lifetime, nutrients can modify physiologic and pathologic processes through epigenetic mechanisms that are critical for gene expression. Modulation of these processes through diet or specific nutrients may prevent diseases and maintain health."[18] This means that following the right diet for our type could help prevent serious illness from developing. That this discovery about how to prevent illness has not made big headlines is unfortunate. Could it be that our society is invested in a health care system that is based on "sick care," rather than prevention (see Chapter 3)? I believe that, once consumers become more aware of the powerful impact of diet on health outcomes, diet and nutrition will become more central to health care in North America.

I ponder on the role of epigenetics in my health. For years, I consumed dairy products with no awareness of my lactose intolerance. In my early 40s, I realized this through experimentation and eliminated cow's milk and its products, but later, at age 57, I was diagnosed with ovarian cancer. I also discovered I have the BRCA2 genetic defect that increases the risk of cancer (breast and ovarian). There is no way to determine the specific impact from the long-term consumption of cow's milk. Given the findings on epigenetics and my sensitivity to milk, I consider it a strong possibility that my years on a wrong diet played a role in activating my defective gene and increased my risk of cancer.

Symptoms of the "Wrong" Diet

The fortunate person may thrive on a variety of foods, while the next person has to keep their diet within a narrow range of options. When seeking your right diet, the traditional diet of your ancestors is an excellent place to start. If your ancestry is unknown or of mixed origins, you can still determine your right diet using bodily symptoms. Your body has an elaborate feedback system that will tell you when your diet is not right, if you understand the body's signals and listen to what they are telling you.

Eating foods unsuited to your needs almost always causes unwanted symptoms, which can vary from person to person, but are remarkably consistent in their meaning. In my clinical experience, I have observed that eating the wrong diet is associated with one or more of the following symptoms:

- Digestive issues–belching, heartburn, gas, abdominal bloating
- Hunger soon after eating
- Cravings for sweet and/or salty foods
- Elimination issues—irregular bowels, constipation, loose stools, frequent or urgent urination
- Mental function—altered mood, irritability, headaches, including migraines
- Respiratory issues—sinus congestion, lung congestion, frequent colds
- Immunity—frequent illness
- Muscles—cramps, achiness
- Joints—stiff, sore
- Skin ailments—rashes, itchiness, and acne breakouts
- Energy—unexplained fatigue, wake up feeling tired, tired after eating
- Sleep disturbances—can't get to sleep, insomnia
- Weight—over or underweight

- Water retention or edema

It is not necessary to have all these symptoms to suspect your diet is not right for you. Some of my clients who were eating the wrong diet experienced only a few of these issues, while others suffered with many. The presence of even a few symptoms is a good reason to reexamine your diet. You may find that your ideal diet is about altering your ratio of proteins, carbohydrates, and fats, or by following a blood type or genotype diet. If you still cannot easily find your ideal diet, you may have allergies or intolerances that are so far undetected. Naturopath Carolee Bateson-Koch warns that ignoring the body's signals that you are eating the wrong diet can lead to serious issues down the road—ulcers, hernias, type 2 diabetes, depression, high blood pressure, obesity, arthritis, and phlebitis.[19]

Allergies, Intolerances, and Sensitivities

Specific foods can cause unwanted reactions in the form of an allergy, intolerance, or sensitivity. These different conditions warrant clarification.

Food allergies result in immediate reactions, such as hives and rapid swelling of the respiratory tract; the latter can be life threatening. Immediate medical treatment is required. Foods to which allergies are common include peanuts and shellfish, but various foods can trigger an allergic response. Because of their severity, allergies are easier to identify, and they show up in medical testing (skin provocation). The causes of allergies are not always known. Canadian authors Lorna Vanderhaeghe and Patrick Bouic point to toxins in the development of allergies with this explanation: "…once the body has reached its limit of toxic load it malfunctions and is unable to distinguish clearly between substances that are not harmful and those that are."[20] When the body does not recognize food as beneficial, the immune system mounts a defense to that food, which we experience as an allergic reaction. Bateson-Koch observes that there are underlying conditions involved in allergies, such as digestive difficulties, mold/fungi and/or parasites.[21] For my clients who have recently developed food allergies, I always investigate these imbalances (see Chapters 11 through 14).

Intolerance to foods represents a reaction that does not involve the immune system in the same way as allergies. For this reason, the skin provocation test used by medical allergy specialists does not detect food intolerances. Celiac disease, for which a medical test exists, is intolerance to gluten found in most grains that produces severe digestive imbalances, weight loss, and overall ill health. Dairy intolerances can be more difficult to identify because they involve the inability to digest one or more components of cow's milk (albumin, casein, whey, or lactose). For some, a total elimination of dairy products is needed. For others, some dairy foods, such as yogurt and cheese, may be tolerated. Those with lactose intolerance are in the latter group. They lack the enzyme lactase, which is needed to digest the milk sugar lactose. The bacterial process involved in making yogurt and cheese turns lactose into lactic acid, which is easier for them to digest.

Lactose intolerance affects approximately 25 percent of the population in North America. According to 2012 statistics in the United States, 75 percent of African-Americans, Jews, Mexican-Americans, and Native Americans, suffer from this intolerance to lactose.[22] A 2010 report by the National Institutes of Health revealed a new discovery; some of those who believe they are lactose intolerant are actually lactose "malabsorbers." The report noted that symptoms of malabsorption will be more difficult to detect.[23]

Sometimes, food intolerances can present very much like allergies. I can attest to the link between my dairy intolerance and allergies. In my twenties, I had respiratory allergies severe enough to require a prescription nasal inhaler. Once I stopped drinking milk, my symptoms were all but eliminated. In my clinical experience, intolerances can produce one or more of the "symptoms of the wrong diet" listed above. This is another way that our biochemical individuality manifests—each person with a food intolerance will present their own symptom pattern.

Sensitivity is a catchall term that refers to allergies and intolerances. I use this term because it includes reactions to non-food items—additives and chemicals. The sensitivities that I identify most often with my clients include dairy, wheat, corn, eggs, soy, nightshade vegetables (tomatoes, potatoes, peppers), and the food additives identified in Chapter 2: aspartame, monosodium glutamate, BHT/BHA, TBHQ, nitrites, sulfites, and artificial food dyes. In my experience, sensitivities to food additives are more common than they were 20 years ago. I believe this is highly related to increased processing of foods and exposure to environmental toxins.

The nature of sensitivities can make them difficult to pinpoint. Some people inherit sensitivities, such as a lack of lactase enzyme to digest lactose in cow's milk. Often sensitivities can develop through life from overeating a food or food group, or after an illness that compromised the digestive tract. Having a small portion of a sensitive food every day is enough to trigger unwanted symptoms. A hard reality is that we may be sensitive to the very foods that we crave. I repeatedly see this with my clients who are sensitive to wheat—they crave breads and cookies. The good news is that there is a systematic approach to identifying or ruling out sensitivities.

Caution: Before investigating sensitivities, you must consult with your medical doctor to rule out illness and disease.

Rule Out Sensitivities

When you have symptoms that point to sensitivities, it is important to identify them as part of determining your right diet. Also, I have developed a systematic method to identify and/or rule out sensitivities to both foods and additives. This method I derived from the elimination diet protocol widely used in holistic nutrition, as well as in my clinical experience.

1.   Recognize symptoms, both past and present

Almost any unwanted symptom represents a malfunction that can relate to a diet unsuited to the individual's needs. Symptoms can even change over time.

One of my clients suffered colic in infancy, respiratory infections as a child, acne as a teenager, and digestive and immune dysfunction as an adult. My assessment determined dairy foods as the trigger for all these symptoms. When he eliminated milk, the symptoms disappeared. As this case illustrates, symptoms do not have to be digestive, and symptom history is important. In addition, because reactions can be subtle or even delayed from 24 to 48 hours, keeping a journal of food and symptoms will help pinpoint possible culprits.

2. Make use of trial diets

Temporary removal of suspected foods is a very effective way to assess their impact. Before doing this, the body must be de-stressed so that you can isolate reactions to specific foods. For this reason, I recommend following the Digestive Balancing Diet (see Appendix 2) for at least 21 days before proceeding to step 3. This trial diet eliminates most of the common sensitive foods and additives.

3. Reintroduce foods in a systematic way

After 21 days on the Digestive Balancing diet, you can start reintroducing foods and substances one at a time to assess their impact. The following represents a self-testing protocol for the most common sensitivities. The key to success lies in the following these instructions in the recommended sequence:

- Continue on the Digestive Balancing Diet.
- Change nothing else about your diet except the substance to be tested.
- Test a new food or substance every four days and note reactions.
- Through the course of testing, substances that prove not to be sensitivities can be re-introduced.
- Foods that produce reactions must be eliminated.
- If there is a reaction, nothing else should be tested for six days. Otherwise the reaction to the first substance can influence the response for the next one.
- Testing is in a defined sequence of foods and substances listed below, starting with those that are more commonly an issue. Additives are tested in the third and fourth months because they have more dramatic effects, making reactions easier to detect.

First month: wheat; cow's milk; nightshade vegetables—tomatoes, potatoes, peppers

Second month: hard cheese; peanuts; soy (e.g., tofu); yeasted bread; mushrooms

Third month: pork; caffeine (e.g., coffee); MSG; aspartame

Fourth month: BHT; sulphites; nitrites; tartrazine; red food dye (one each week)

- On the day a food is to be tested, one meal comprises that food alone. For example, if testing wheat, eat a big plate of pasta or two slices of sourdough bread (note: yeasted breads are tested separately). If dairy is being tested, have a big glass of cow's milk. Watch for any adverse responses from those listed under "Symptoms of the Wrong Diet" earlier in this chapter. For testing additives, have a large portion of food that contains the additive. Chapter 2 provides the food sources for additives.

- Responses can occur immediately or up to 48 hours following a test.
- A food journal is helpful to track reactions to foods/substances.

4. You might need help

Step 3 may seem onerous and time consuming, or perhaps after going through steps 1 through 3, you are still unsure of your sensitivities. Multiple sensitivities can make it difficult to isolate the offenders. Many holistic practitioners have reliable tests for sensitivities, such as applied kinesiology, galvanic skin response, RAST, and blood tests. In my practice, I use the galvanic skin response testing, specifically the Bioenergetic Evaluation (see Appendix 1). This proven method, in use for over 50 years, involves measuring the energy response to foods and additives. It bears repeating that the skin provocation test used by medical allergy specialists identifies allergies but not sensitivities to either foods or additives.

Your Right Diet

Eating the right diet is the foundation for good health and for the prevention of illness. Remedies of any kind, drugs, or supplements, will not make up for a diet that does not meet your individual needs. Finding your right diet is a personal quest, not a prescriptive one-size-fits-all program. You may tolerate a wide variety of foods, in which case the previous chapter, Quality Food and Toxin-Free Living, will support your health goals. Some individuals may thrive on a vegetarian diet, while others fare better as meat eaters. You may find that eating too many carbohydrates causes imbalances in blood sugar, a condition associated with cravings for sugary foods and often weight gain. If you have any of the symptoms I describe in this chapter, it is critical to rule out sensitivities to both foods and additives.

I must emphasize that multiple sensitivities often go hand in hand with imbalances in the digestive tract. Malfunction in digestion, absorption, or elimination can result from eating the Standard American Diet (SAD), from infectious agents (viruses, bacteria, and parasites), or environmental toxins. In this situation, sensitivities to foods and additives *result* from dietary choices or infections, and sometimes both. Because the SAD is nutritionally deficient, there is a higher risk of succumbing to an infection. Restoring health in such instances depends on therapeutic holistic interventions covered in Part 3 of this book.

Issues with food are also intricately connected with our emotional balance. The next chapter outlines the mental/emotional aspects involved in the quest for being well.

Chapter Notes

1. "Holistic Nutrition Scope of Practice," *Canadian School of Natural Nutrition,* accessed June 10, 2014, www.csnn.ca/holistic-nutrition-industry/.

2. Michael Pollan, *In Defense of Food: An Eater's Manifesto* (New York, New York: Penguin Press, 2008).

3. United States, Department of Health and Human Services, National Institutes of Health, "Lactose Intolerance," *National Digestive Diseases Information Clearinghouse (NDDIC),* accessed June 10, 2014, http://digestive.niddk.nih.gov/ddiseases/pubs/lactoseintolerance/#risk.

4. Michael Pollan, *In Defense of Food.*

5. Roger J. Williams, PhD, *Biochemical Individuality: The Basis for the Genotrophic Concept* (New Canaan, Connecticut: Keats Publishing, 1998).

6. Dr. Johanna Budwig, *Flax Oil as a True Aid against Arthritis, Heart Infarction, Cancer and Other Diseases* (Vancouver, B.C.: Apple Publishing Co., 1992).

7. Colin T. Campbell, PhD and Thomas M. Campbell II, *The China Study: Startling Implications for Diet, Weight Loss and Long-Term Health* (Dallas, Texas: Benbella Books, 2006).

8. Ibid., 85.

9. Robert C. Atkins, MD, *Dr. Atkins' New Diet Revolution: The Amazing No-Hunger Weight-Loss Plan That Has Helped Millions Lose Weight and Keep it Off* (New York, New York: Avon Books, 1992).

10. Gary Foster et al., "Weight and Metabolic Outcomes after 2 Years on a Low-Carbohydrate versus Low-Fat Diet: A Randomized Trial," *Annals of Internal Medicine* 153 no.3 (2010): 147-157, accessed June 10, 2014, http://www.ncbi.nlm.nih.gov/pubmed/20679559.

11. F. Hu, J. Manson and W. Willet, "Types of Dietary Fat and Risk of Coronary Heart Disease: A Critical Review," *Journal of American College of Nutrition* 20 (2001): 5-19, accessed June 11, 2014, http://www.ncbi.nlm.nih.gov/pubmed/11293467.

12. Colin T. Campbell PhD and Thomas M. Campbell II, *The China Study.*

13. Luigi Fontana et al., "Long-term low-protein, low-calorie diet and endurance exercise modulate metabolic factors associated with cancer risk," *American Journal of Clinical Nutrition* 84 no.6 (2006): 1456-1462, accessed June 11, 2014, http://www.ncbi.nlm.nih.gov/pubmed/17158430.

14. William L. Wollcott and Trish Fahey, *The Metabolic Typing Diet: Customize Your Diet for: Permanent Weight Loss, Optimal Health, Preventing and Reversing Disease, Staying Young at Any Age* (New York, New York: Broadway Books, 2000).

15. Dr. Joseph Mercola, "Nutritional Typing Articles," *Mercola.com,* accessed October 20, 2014, http://nutritionaltype.mercola.com/.

16. Dr. Peter J. D'Adamo, *Eat Right for Your Type* (New York, New York: Berkeley Publishing Group, 2002).

17. ___. *Change Your Genetic Destiny* (New York, New York: Broadway Books, 2007), 117.

18. Sang-woon Choi and Simonetta Friso, "Epigenetics: A New Bridge between Nutrition and Health," *Advances in Nutrition* 1 (November 2010), accessed October 21, 2014, doi: 10.3945/an.110.1004.

19. Carolee Bateson-Koch, DC, ND, *Allergies: Disease in Disguise: How to Heal Your Allergic Condition Permanently and Naturally* (Burnaby, British Columbia: Alive Books, 1994), 44-5.

20. Lorna Vanderhaeghe and Patrick Bouic, *The Immune System Cure: Nature's Way to Super-Powered Health* (Toronto, Ontario: Prentice Hall Canada: 1999), 157.

21. Carolee Bateson-Koch, DC, ND, *Allergies: Disease in Disguise.*

22. "Lactose Intolerance Statistics," *National Digestive Diseases Information* (July 23, 2012) accessed August 11, 2014, www.statisticbrain.com/lactose-intolerance-statistics/.

23. United States, Department of Health and Human Services, National Institutes of Health, "Lactose Intolerance and Health," *NIH Consensus Development Conference,* February 22-24, 2010, accessed August 20, 2014, http://consensus.nih.gov/2010/lactose.htm.

9: BALANCED EMOTIONS, BALANCED HEALTH

In Chapter 6, I discuss how emotional states affect health, both positively and negatively. To be completely well, we may have to work on our emotional balance. Unfortunately, our emotional *im*balances can go unnoticed or even rationalized—*that's just the way I am* or *I'm just like my mother/father*—that is, until we face a health crisis. It is then that emotional balance becomes so critical to healing, as I discovered:

In 2010, I was diagnosed with ovarian cancer and the doctors told me that if I did not take chemotherapy and radiation, I would be dead in three years. As surprising as it may seem, I do not remember being overcome with fear. Instead, I said, "This is interesting. I wonder what I will learn from this." I had already spent several years focusing on my emotional, social, spiritual, and psychological balance—and I believe that this grounding helped me handle "the Big C" diagnosis. More importantly, I could examine how my past emotional response patterns may have had a role in the development of cancer. At times, I even feel grateful for the experience because it crystallized what, prior to my diagnosis, had been an academic understanding of how emotional balance contributes to being well. I learned firsthand about the power of positive thoughts, spiritual practice, and energy healing.

In this chapter, I offer what I have learned from helping people in my career in social work and holistic nutrition, as well as my personal quest for emotional balance. Seeking emotional balance starts with an awareness of what we need to change. I submit this; no one is perfectly balanced emotionally. I offer three areas for self-assessment of emotional balance:

Emotional relationships to food
Emotional responses to people and situations
Beliefs that can affect health

Emotional Relationships to Food

Our relationship with food can be complicated. Besides providing nourishment, food evokes emotional reactions: fun, camaraderie with others, and even comfort. While it is okay to take pleasure from eating, there is a point at which food can become an emotional prop, commonly known as "emotional eating" or "comfort eating." I seldom hear of anyone turning to *healthy* foods for comfort. Emotional attachments are usually for sweets, such as ice cream, cookies, chips, chocolate bars, but sometimes salty foods like chips. It is no coincidence that these foods are carbohydrates that provide quick energy, and for some, a boost in mood. The nature of these high-glycemic "carbs" is a rapid rise in blood sugar, soon followed by a rapid drop accompanied by fatigue, or depressed mood. Overeating sweets and starchy foods will make such symptoms worse. People who experience these symptoms regularly should see a medical doctor to be assessed for diabetes.

Foods can become an obsession bordering on addiction. In this state, the focus is on food's emotional benefits instead of its nutritional ones—*living to eat* instead of *eating to live*. It is important to note that food cravings may also be a symptom of a physiological imbalance. Many of my clients come to me believing they are doomed to live with food cravings, only to see them disappear with diet changes and/or a healing protocol. Before concluding that attachments to food are purely emotional, it is critical to ensure that your diet is right for your needs (see Chapter 8) and rule out other sources of cravings such as food sensitivities and blood sugar imbalances (see Chapter 11 and 14). If these food connections are resolved, you are ready to investigate emotional attachments to food.

To examine emotional relationships with food requires a critical look at your eating habits and attitudes toward food. Answering "yes" to the following questions points to unhealthy relationships with food:

Do I feel the necessity to snack on junk food while watching TV or relaxing?

Are there foods that I feel drawn to when feeling down or stressed?

Do I crave sweets, chocolate, or salty snacks to where I make a special trip to the store for them?

Do I have one food that I consider my "comfort" food?

If you struggle with weight, it is helpful to ask yourself these questions:

Do I fear eating food, even healthy food, because I am afraid of gaining weight?

Do I feel guilty after eating certain foods? (e.g., fats, sweets)

Worry and guilt about giving in to forbidden foods can be as destructive as eating them. In *The Slow Down Diet*, Marc David cites evidence that worrying about dietary fat and overweight can promote weight gain. Anxiety about food and eating can cause our bodies to store fat instead of burn it.[1]

Emotional Responses to People and Situations

The work of David Hawkins, discussed in Chapter 6, determined that some emotions are health supportive: courage, trust, optimism, forgiveness, understanding, love, and joy. Conversely, the emotions of pride, anger, desire, fear, grief, apathy, guilt, and shame are physically weakening. Therefore, it is critical to recognize how much these emotions are at play. If you are not sure how predominant negative feelings are, answering these questions provide clues:

How many times a day do I criticize others or myself? The more frequently this is, the higher the likelihood that lower energy emotions are predominant.

How many negative comments or criticisms do I make in a day? This behaviour pattern can eventually adversely affect physical health.

Do people react to me negatively? Responses from others can mirror what we have given them.

If answers to these questions point to a negative emotional pattern, the following question becomes relevant:

Do I suffer from ailments that respond poorly to treatment/therapies? Negative emotions can block healing.

There is a risk in acknowledging our negative emotional patterns. Accepting responsibility for unhealthy emotions in creating our health problems can be another blow to an already fragile emotional state. Feeling guilty that we made ourselves sick will not help either. If you are now worrying about the impact of your own negative thoughts and feelings, Carolyn Myss, a renowned medical intuitive, provides hope: "We all have negative feelings, but not all negativity produces disease. To create disease, negative emotions have to be dominant, and what accelerates the process is *knowing* the negative thought to be toxic but giving it permission to thrive in your consciousness anyway."[2]

Beliefs That Can Affect Health

Without realizing it, we perceive events according to our personal beliefs about the world and ourselves. We form such beliefs through our lives by learning from all our experiences. Messages we hear, our parent's attitudes, the culture in which we live, come together to create our "world view"—a lens through which we interpret events and experiences. For instance, people who grow up in a war-torn country may view the world as threatening. This view can cause them to perceive new experiences more fearfully than those raised in a peaceful country. Living in fear is not health supportive. In this way, our beliefs influence our physical health.

Some beliefs about the self can have negative health effects. Louise Hay outlines the most damaging ones, which she calls "limiting beliefs"—views about ourselves that can be detrimental to our health and happiness. Hay identifies three limiting beliefs I observe often with my clients who have nagging health issues:

I'm not good enough

Life is dangerous

Lack of self-love[3]

Let us further explore these three self-limiting beliefs.

Most of us have a belief about not being good enough at *something*, which is not all that limiting. After all, we must be realistic about our abilities. That is not the issue; it is when we think we are not good at *anything* that our emotional state can have negative physical consequences. To assess your belief about being good enough, ask yourself this question:

Do I avoid trying something new for fear of embarrassment? Do I stop trying for fear of failure? This can point to a belief that you are "not good enough."

Believing life is dangerous can manifest as phobias (e.g., fear of open spaces, fear of heights) or hold us back from taking risks in life. However, this can also save us from taking unnecessary risks. I have no desire to go skydiving because I believe it is an unnecessary risk for the sake of a few moments' thrill. A certain amount of caution about dangers in the world is justified. It is when fears dominate our thoughts and actions that they become threats to health. To determine how dominant fear is for you, ask yourself:

Do I hold fears that others consider unreasonable or unfounded? This can indicate unhealthy beliefs.

Lack of self-love often translates into the belief that we are not worthy of love from others as in, "no one loves me." Feelings of self-loathing, in the extreme, can cause self-destructive behaviours (e.g., drinking alcohol to excess, overeating). Eating disorders such as anorexia and bulimia can develop out of severe cases of self-loathing. Many of us have something we dislike about ourselves—a big nose, overweight, bad skin. Does this mean that we believe we are unlovable? Not necessarily. At what point does this have the potential to affect physical health? Answering the following questions with "yes" is a sign that this limiting belief has a potentially negative health effect:

Do I have trouble getting along with one or more co-workers or close relatives? Has this happened more than once in my life?

Do I have trouble maintaining loving relationships?

Unfortunately, lack of self-love can make us less loving towards others and then discourages others from giving us the love that we desire. In this way, a limiting belief becomes a self-fulfilling prophecy.

On the upside, beliefs in positive outcomes can be a source for being well. There is some evidence our ability to heal from illness may be based more on belief than on the medicines we take. In *The Biology of Belief: Unleashing the Power of Consciousness, Matter & Miracles*, Dr. Bruce Lipton states, "In more than half of the clinical trials for the six leading antidepressants, the drugs did not outperform the placebo or sugar pills."[4] The placebo is a well-known phenomenon in which the belief in a remedy makes a difference to healing. Dr. Bernie Siegel has documented cases of healing from cancer among patients who believed they were taking a medicine that was actually a placebo. To some people these healing seemed miraculous, but it clearly illustrates the power of belief and expectation.[5] The placebo effect illustrates the power of belief to effect healing. On the other hand, a lack of belief in a treatment or therapy can make illness worse and even hasten death.

I am particularly struck by the discovery of Dr. Bruce Lipton, a renowned genetics researcher who came to realize the power that beliefs have over health. Based on his research, he had to discount his own field of study and conclude that DNA was *not* the determinant of health, as he had once believed. This was so challenging to prevailing genetics theories that Dr. Lipton's colleagues ostracized him. Despite threats to his career, he stood by his position: "belief controls biology."[6]

Lipton's revelation is significant; it provides hope for being well, if we can ensure our beliefs are health supportive.

With greater awareness of limiting beliefs, as well as emotional relationships with food, family and friends, it is easier to identify the change(s) needed to promote emotional balance. Based on my personal and clinical experience, I have identified eight principles for establishing a health-supportive emotional balance. These principles are about choices we can make in our personal, social, and spiritual life. They are interrelated; some are foundations for other principles. Emotional balance is more likely to come through attention to all these principles with the realization that this could be a lifelong quest. As Ralph Waldo Emerson said, "Life is a journey, not a destination."

Eight Principles for Emotional Balance

1. Take responsibility for health and healing

A foundational principle is that of taking personal responsibility for our health-related activities. Too many of us have given responsibility for our health to practitioners whom we expect to *cure* us. In contrast, with a holistic approach, we are active participants in our own health and healing. In the presence of illness, this means that we become aware of how we got sick in the first place and proceed in solution mode. I have found this affirmation by Carolyn Myss to be helpful: "I am responsible for the creation of my health. I participated at some level in the creation of this illness. I can participate in the healing of this illness by healing myself…my emotional, psychological, physical and spiritual being."[7] It is important not to play a blame game. Some of our actions are rooted in experiences the memory of which we stored in our subconscious because they are too painful. Often, we are not aware of the negative energy such memories have exerted on our bodies. It is more important to make an honest appraisal of our emotional connections to make changes in the present. As Dr. Bernie Siegel aptly puts it: "People have the built-in potential to induce self-healing."[8] I believe we can promote self-healing by applying the other seven principles offered here.

2. Surround yourself with supportive people

"Marry the right person," states H. Jackson Brown, in his *21 Suggestions for Success,* "this one decision will determine 90% of our happiness or misery."[9] Equally important are the people with whom we choose to associate in our work and social circles. Being around positive, uplifting, and supportive people is health giving. Negative people subject us to lower energies that will bring us down, both physically and psychologically. The decision to seek more health-supportive relationships could mean that some friends do not fit well anymore. I am not recommending quitting friendships because I believe any relationship can change if we start responding to that person with forgiveness and love (see Principles 6 and 7).

In choosing our associations and community groups, the ones with missions that inspire or uplift us will naturally connect us to supportive people. We may lament the high rate of divorce, but it can also be a sign that people are less willing to stick it out in unsupportive relationships. I have been happily married for over 30 years, to the same person, but my husband had been divorced from his first wife. She is also remarried, and happily so. Their decision to leave their unsupportive relationship has made all the difference to the emotional balance of four individuals.

3. Serve others

Only a life lived for others is worthwhile ~ Albert Einstein

Emotional balance is easier when we are fulfilled in what we do. I agree with Einstein; the ultimate fulfillment comes from making a difference in the lives of others. I know that not all careers allow us to do that, but in any job, we can have a serving attitude toward those with whom we work. If this is not sufficient, there are many volunteer opportunities to allow such fulfillment.

Serving is about giving of ourselves, but there is an unfortunate attitude that if we give of ourselves too much, we will lose something. Many faith traditions espouse the belief that it is in giving that we receive the most. This may be difficult to believe, but the best way to overcome a fear of giving is to do it and watch what happens. Any volunteer work that I have ever done has always given me much more in return. We do not give in order to receive something, but it will happen anyway. Some of the most revered and inspiring public figures gave of themselves unconditionally, for example Mother Teresa and Nelson Mandela. It is not necessary to make the level of sacrifices these two did; but we can all do something. This was dramatically portrayed in the book and feature film, *Pay it Forward,* in which people helped others because they were asked to pass on the help they themselves had received. The outcomes for the givers, some of whom were homeless and drug-addicted, were life changing.[10] Although this story was fictional, I believe it to be a true-to-life depiction of how serving others benefit the givers.

4. Learn from mistakes

There is the saying that we learn more from our mistakes than from our successes. This can go as far as celebrating mistakes because of the lessons they offer us. Unfortunately, many of us dwell on past mistakes, to the point of inducing guilt and shame. Why do we make mistakes, or worse, make the same mistakes repeatedly? I subscribe to Marianne Williamson's view in her book *The Gift of Change: Spiritual Guidance for Living Your Best Life*: "Every mistake we ever made occurred because at the moment we made it we were not in conscious contact with our highest self."[11] When I read this, I had to admit that most of my mistakes came from focusing on my own interests, not my higher, altruistic self. Check this out yourself. After a mistake, explore the feelings related to it. *Were you interested in the needs of all concerned or in your own needs or wants?* If we are aware of the motivation for mistakes, we are less likely to repeat them.

Guilt over mistakes is a destructive emotion that inhibits healing. With respect to illness, we may feel guilty about past poor health habits that triggered our illness.

This is not health promoting. An illness is best viewed as a wake-up call to make needed changes or to learn more about ourselves. I can attest to this. While going through surgery and treatment for cancer, I came to understand that, besides a reminder to take better care of myself, there were serendipities from the experience—more compassion for others, greater humility, and the strength that comes from faith in a higher power.

5. Decide to be happy

Happiness is when what you think, what you say, and what you do are in harmony. ~ Mahatma Gandhi

Being happy is health supportive. A 2003 study published in the *British Journal of Nursing* identified how happy emotions can relate to physical health. Participants with happy emotions exhibited a greater ability to fight off colds than those who were unhappy.[12] While we know being happy will help us feel better, the dilemma is in knowing *how* to be happy.

It is easy to be caught up in thinking that happiness is based on what we have or what we achieve, and we are not alone. The prevailing North American belief is that happiness comes from material gain and success. This is depicted in the film *The Pursuit of Happyness,* a portrayal of one man's hard-won success in the corporate world, which he equates with happiness.[13] In contrast, *Happy,* a 2011 documentary film, explored happiness across different cultures and found that the happiest people were often those who had the least material wealth.[14] These opposing views on the sources of happiness can cause emotional stress because we do not know which to believe.

I believe that, despite societal messages, happiness is not based on power, wealth, or fame. Seeking happiness through accomplishments or material possessions will always leave us wanting more, because there is always more to have. Happiness comes from peace with ourselves and with others, and this is a daily decision we can make, regardless of our situation. In *The Gift of Change: Spiritual Guidance for Living Your Best Life*, Marianne Williamson says this well: "There are always things to be happy about and there are always things to be sad about. The bridge to a happier life is a more emotional decision than a change in circumstance."[15]

When there are truly tragic events, we will find our happiness understandably disrupted for a time. However, we can avoid prolonged unhappiness by taking a long view of the situation. Some of the most inspiring stories of the human condition come from those who can smile in the face of imminent death. Have they discovered the secret to true happiness? During my bout with cancer, I learned about my resilience and the caring of family and friends, which gave me reasons to celebrate. I was pleasantly surprised to find things to be happy about amid a personal trial.

One helpful strategy during a personal trial is to choose activities that make us laugh. As a long-time feature in the *Readers Digest* says, "Laughter is the best medicine." Based on his clinical experience, Dr. Bernie Siegel maintains that laughter aids in healing even the worst illnesses, such as cancer. Laughter invokes positive feelings and energy that can promote healing. At the physiological level, laughter releases chemicals that support the immune system. So, when suffering with an illness, it can help to seek opportunities to laugh. This also means not paying too much attention to the news, which is primarily about tragic events. It is a sad fact that bad news sells more than happy news. As a culture, we seem to afford laughter little value, and it shows in our entertainment. Since the inception of the Academy Awards, I identified only one winner for Best Picture that was billed as a comedy— *Annie Hall* in 1977. Notably, even this film's had some tragic elements. Being able to laugh every day is emotionally and physically beneficial. We can associate with people who make us laugh, read comic strips, learn a few clean jokes, or watch comedic entertainment.

6. Practice forgiveness

When you judge another, you do not define them; you define yourself. ~ Wayne W. Dyer

Lack of forgiveness will literally eat away at the body and the spirit. The ability to forgive others and ourselves is therefore critical to health. *A Course in Miracles,* a curriculum for spiritual transformation, links physical health directly to forgiveness with this statement: "For no one in whom true forgiveness rests can suffer... [The person] who forgives is healed."[16]

True forgiveness is difficult. In a world where blame, fault finding and legal litigation are commonplace, and even applauded, how do we become more forgiving? After all, we cannot look the other way when people commit crimes. Justice is at the core of a civilized society in which unacceptable behaviour cannot be condoned. In answer to these challenges, I find Louise Hay's perspective on forgiveness very helpful: "We need to understand that whoever we need most to forgive was also in pain...they were doing the best they could with the understanding, awareness, and knowledge they had at that time."[17] In this statement, I see two keys to developing true forgiveness—more compassion and less criticism. Karen Armstrong's *12 Steps to a Compassionate Life* offers a step-by-step process for developing a more compassionate and forgiving spirit. Armstrong also launched a worldwide movement called the Charter for Compassion. In his book, *A Complaint-Free World,* Will Bowen offers a spiritual yet practical guide for reducing our all-too-common habit of criticizing others and ourselves.

7. Focus on love, not fear

All you need is love. ~ John Lennon and Paul McCartney

It is unfortunate that this iconic Beatles lyric from the 1960s has yet to result in the belief that love is *really* all we need. *A Course in Miracles,* which I have studied since 2009, teaches that there are only two emotions: love and fear. Unfortunately, for most of us, fear predominates our thinking and, because we live in a fear-based society, this is often without our conscious awareness. Fear of other countries, cultures, and religions is often what binds us together both nationally and culturally. I observe that governments and businesses often base their decisions on fear that another country or corporation will gain the upper hand. Again, I turn to entertainment to illustrate the central place of fear in our lives. Most of the movie blockbusters are about some real or imagined fear. War films chronicle actual fearful events, but imagined fears—vampires, alien invasions, and end-of the world scenarios—are box office hits. It seems we have a perverse attraction to being fearful, and this becomes our emotional lens for viewing events and other people's actions. The more fearful we are, the more fear we experience.

It takes a tremendous amount of spiritual discipline to seek and give love in the midst of our fear-based society. However, I believe it is possible to learn how to shift from a focus on fear to loving others and ourselves. We have a choice—we can decide to look for love in all situations. Nurturing this choice will depend on embracing other principles offered here, such as practicing forgiveness and deciding to be happy.

Having a regular spiritual practice or a spiritual perspective is critical to make loving responses predominate over fearful ones. In the New Testament (NIV), 1 John 4:18 states: "There is no fear in love. But perfect love drives out fear, because fear has to do with punishment. The one who fears is not made perfect in love." *A Course in Miracles* makes a clear connection between emotional and physical healing with this declaration: "all healing involves replacing fear with love."[18] One of the most important lessons I have learned from *A Course in Miracles* is that what we perceive as an "attack" from someone else is in reality their call for love. This understanding makes it easier to love others, even those who we consider an enemy. Insight on how to have a more loving perspective can also be found in books by Marianne Williamson, Wayne Dyer, Louise Hay, Deepak Chopra, and Eckhart Tolle.

8. Realize you are not alone

Begin to see yourself as a soul with a body rather than a body with a soul. ~ Wayne W. Dyer

We are spiritual beings at one with an infinitely powerful Source that may be called God or Divine Spirit. The name we give to the Source depends on our personal spiritual philosophy. Many scientists and quantum physicists now accept the existence of a universal energy source, so this is no longer merely a religious or spiritual tenet. I find it helpful to think of Source like a radio signal. By tuning in and listening to Source, we receive guidance for our good and for the good of others. Staying tuned in is the challenge. We have static interference from the world, and we can increase this interference when we focus too much on our individual interests. This is an instance when belief in oneself can be as destructive as having too little belief. Too much belief in ourselves as the master of our fate belies the reliance we have on Source for our ultimate spiritual strength. Self-help author and motivational speaker Wayne Dyer likens us to a drop of water in the ocean. Our full potential is only realized when we as individuals (drops of water) recognize that we are one with our Source (the ocean). When we see ourselves as separate from our Source—as only a drop of water—we lose connection with our full potential for joy and love.[19]

When we tune in to Source, we can marshal the healing energies we need for both emotional and physical well-being. Authors in energy and spiritual healing, such as Dr. Bernie Siegel, Carolyn Myss, and Deepak Chopra, recognize that seemingly miraculous healings come from this connection to Source. By accepting we are connected with our Source, we realize we are all connected to each other—in our oneness with Source. Once we embrace this truth, it means that blaming, condemning, or attacking anyone else amounts to blaming, condemning, and attacking ourselves. In these states, we cannot heal either emotionally or physically. The other principles I have discussed come into play. When we accept our connection to Source and each other, only love and forgiveness for others and ourselves make sense. Happiness is the resulting emotional state. Serving others becomes second nature.

Being at one with Source may seem difficult to achieve. Its ultimate expression, spiritual enlightenment, is widely believed to be the achievement of a select few—Jesus, Buddha, Mohammed. But many people have spiritual insights, such as intuition, extrasensory perception, and clairvoyance. Others report receiving answers to prayer. Even if you have not experienced these phenomena, most of us have had a glimpse of them in what seems to be just a coincidence. Have you ever thought of someone you have not talked to in a while, and a few minutes later, they call you on the phone? I believe this is what can happen when we tune into Source, and each other. To me, this small *miracle* means it is also possible to experience *miraculous* healing from serious illness.

Of the eight principles for emotional balance presented here, accepting and applying the principle that "we are not alone" is perhaps the most difficult. In this brief précis of a complex issue, I aim to inspire you to seek the connection with Source, realizing that this will probably involve lifelong study and practice.

The Quest for Emotional Balance

How you feel today results from the various experiences, thoughts, feelings, and beliefs that you hold now and have held in the past. Awareness of which of these areas are affecting your health is a critical first step. Embracing the emotionally supportive principles that I offer here is the next step. You may find it best to focus on a few principles at a time—some will be of more help to you than others. Your transformation will depend on your personal commitment to thinking, perceiving, believing, and acting in ways that are health supportive.

There are different approaches and tools you can use to reduce negative emotions and harness the power of positive ones, such as affirmations,[20] meditation, yoga, journaling, prayer, spiritual study, counseling, energy work (e.g., Emotional Freedom Technique[21]), intuitive healing, and dream analysis. For me, spiritual study, meditation, and prayer make a critical difference. Lynne McTaggart, in her book *The Intention Experiment: Using Your Thoughts to Change Your Life and the World,* reports on the many studies that demonstrate the power of prayer and intention.[22] It really helps to ask people to pray for us or send healing thoughts, particularly if prayers or thoughts are specific and focused. The tools or approaches that work for you will depend on your philosophy, personality and learning style.

Learning styles differ. We learn best in one of three ways: tactile, auditory, or visual. This can influence what approach works best in our journey to emotional balance. A tactile person can benefit emotionally from yoga or EFT. For an auditory learner, the ideal might be reciting affirmations, listening to guided meditation, or hearing how others have healed themselves in a support group. Visual learners would gain more emotional support from nature or art (e.g., drawing, painting, crafts, sculpting), or from reading inspirational or educational books. We may have some of each learning style, but with one more predominant, in particular for emotionally charged issues. If you are not sure of your predominant learning style, consider the words you would use when giving an opinion on something of importance. Tactile learners might say, "I feel…;" auditory learners, "I think…;" and visual learners, "I see…"

Our body's physical status, and capacity for being well, is closely tied to our emotional state. But, we are mortal beings; we cannot will ourselves to live forever. Our attitudes towards life and death must also be balanced. Dr. Bernie Siegel gives us this profound thought: "Getting well is not the only goal. Even more important is learning to love without fear, to be at peace with life and ultimately, death. Then healing can occur and one is no longer set up for failure (by believing one can cure all physical problems and never die)."[23]

I have a profound experience facing my potential demise after a cancer diagnosis. While going through cancer surgery and treatments, I did not pray, "Please, God, save my life." This was my prayer: "If I have more to achieve in this existence, please grace me with physical healing." Because I knew I would have an answer to this prayer, it brought me untold peace.

Chapter Notes

1. Marc David, *The Slow Down Diet: Eating for Pleasure, Energy & Weight Loss* (Rochester, Vermont: Healing Arts Press, 2005).

2. Carolyn Myss, PhD, *Anatomy of the Spirit: The Seven Stages of Power and Healing* (New York, New York: Three Rivers Press, 1996), 43.

3. Louise Hay, *You Can Heal Your Life* (Carlsbad, California: Hay House, 1999), 42-3.

4. Bruce H. Lipton, PhD, *The Biology of Belief: Unleashing the Power of Consciousness, Matter & Miracles* (Santa Rosa, California: Mountain of Love/Elite Books, 2005), 141.

5. Bernie S. Siegel, MD, *Love, Medicine and Miracles: Lessons Learned about Self-Healing from a Surgeon's Experience with Exceptional Patients* (New York, New York: Harper & Row, 1986.

6. Bruce H. Lipton, PhD, *The Biology of Belief*.

7. Carolyn Myss, PhD, *Anatomy of the Spirit,* 47.

8. Bernie Siegel, MD, *The Art of Healing: Uncovering Your Inner Wisdom and Potential for Self-Healing* (Novato, California: New World Library, 2013), 8.

9. H. Jackson Brown, Jr., *21 Suggestions for Success,* accessed April 20, 2014, http://web.utk.edu/~jgoverly/21suggestions.html.

10. Ryan Hyde, *Pay it Forward* (New York: Simon & Shuster, 2000); *Pay it Forward,* DVD, directed by Mimi Leder, (Los Angeles, California: Warner Bros., 2000). In this book/film, "paying it forward" means doing something to help three people and asking nothing in return except that they, in turn, do something to help three other people.

11. Marianne Williamson, *The Gift of Change: Spiritual Guidance for a Radically New Life* (San Francisco: Harper Books, 2004), 73.

12. Janine Jones, "Stress response, pressure ulcer development and adaptation," *British Journal of Nursing* 12 no.2 (2003, on-line September 27, 2013): 17-23, accessed September 6, 2014, http://dx.doi.org/10.12968/bjon.2003.12.Sup2.11321.

13. *The Pursuit of Happyness,* DVD, directed by Gabriel Muccino (Hollywood, California: Columbia Pictures, 2006).

14. *Happy,* DVD, directed by Roko Belic (San Jose, California: Iris Films, 2011).

15. Marianne Williamson, *The Gift of Change,* 48.

16. *A Course in Miracles, Combined Volume, Workbook,* Third Edition (Mill Valley, California: Foundation for Inner Peace, 2007), 569.

17. Louise Hay, *You Can Heal Your Life,* 22.

18. *A Course in Miracles,* Workbook, 158.

19. Wayne W. Dyer, *There's a Spiritual Solution to Every Problem* (California: HarperCollins Publishers, 2003).

20. Louise Hay, *You Can Heal Your Life.*

21. Gary Flint, PhD, *Emotional Freedom: Techniques for Dealing with Physical and Emotional Distress* (Vernon, British Columbia: NeoSolTerric Enterprises, 2001).

22. Lynne McTaggart, *The Intention Experiment: Using Your Thoughts to Change Your Life and the World* (New York, New York: Free Press, 2007).

23. Bernie S. Siegel, MD, *Love, Medicine and Miracles,* 42.

PART 3: HOLISTIC GUIDES FOR RESTORING HEALTHY BALANCE

This part is primarily for those who already suffer from nagging symptoms or health conditions and want to use a natural healing approach. The prerequisites to applying this information are in Part 2: Holistic Guides to Being Well. Once there are health issues, however, following these guides may not be enough to restore health. Holistic nutrition practice has assessment processes and healing protocols to restore good health. First, it is essential to know how natural healing works (Chapter 10). Next, there must be an understanding of the body's signals of poor function (Chapter 11). The remaining chapters detail the proven interventions I have used to help my clients restore their health.

Rather than presenting a series of prescriptive protocols, I offer a template for healing based on my Holistic Model of Wellness, which considers individual responses to diet and environment. The process of restoring healthy function must be based on your individual situation. This is not meant to be vague; it reflects the reality that natural healing must be customized to your needs. One-size-fits-all protocols do not work! Using a holistic healing template, you can restore healthy balance, address physical deterioration, and reduce the risk of illness. My message is one of hope: Almost anyone has the capacity to be well.

You will not find protocols for diagnosed medical conditions and illnesses because that is the medical approach. Before applying the recommendations in this part of the book, it is important to rule out serious illness through consultation with a medical doctor. If there is no diagnosable illness, any remaining health issues are apt to relate to how the body is functioning, for which there are holistic and natural healing solutions.

10: UNDERSTAND NATURAL HEALING

The physician treats, but nature heals. ~ Hippocrates

Often, our best efforts to support good health will still result in an illness or health condition. Thankfully, our bodies have natural healing powers that are highly evolved and effective, though sometimes slower than we would like. In today's society, there is an impatient attitude that tempts us to take shortcuts to healing with medications. While drugs may relieve symptoms, they are neither natural nor do they promote true healing. Natural healing is rooted in the body's innate desire for homeostasis, defined as *the ability or tendency of an organism or cell to maintain internal equilibrium by adjusting its physiological processes*. A state of homeostasis means there is balanced function among all body systems: circulation, respiration, blood sugar, hormones, immunity, digestion, elimination, nervous system, and cell metabolism. When our bodies are out of balance, it is important to know that certain activities support healing while others block it. To engage the body's natural healing processes, we need to understand how they work and how best to support them.

Why We Get Sick

You might well ask: *If the body is so good at healing, why do we become ill?* In Part 1, I outline the challenges to being well: nutrient-deficient food, food additives, viruses, bacteria, parasites, environmental toxins, injury, and emotional stress. I call these life stressors and health events, and if there are too many, the body's homeostasis will be upset and health will suffer. The process of going from well to unwell is depicted in Figure 2: The Path to Being Unwell. The Xs marked along the top represent life stressors and health events, e.g., emotional experiences, physical illness, or injury. The last stressor/event on the right of the model becomes the last straw when homeostasis is upset. At that point, health status declines, often dramatically. Sudden loss of health may appear to relate to the last stressor/event, but illness is always the cumulative result of everything that has happened. Here are some specific examples of health events and life stressors that contribute to the loss of homeostasis:

- Eating a poor quality diet, e.g., foods high in refined sugars/grains, trans fats
- Eating a diet that is wrong for individual needs
- Bacterial infections—both acute and chronic, e.g., root canals can be chronically infected, which depresses the immune system response
- Viral infections—both acute and chronic, e.g., Epstein Barr, a common virus, can be a lingering infection linked with chronic fatigue syndrome

- Parasitic infections—damage the digestive tract, which impairs nutrient absorption
- Toxic overload from heavy metals or chemicals
- Death of a loved one
- Divorce
- Loss of employment
- Physical injury
- Using medications and supplements to control symptoms

Once homeostasis is lost, some form of illness will manifest, and following the Holistic Guides to Being Well (Part 2) may not be enough to restore balanced function. Therapeutic interventions may be required and, to be effective, they must work *with* the body's natural healing process. The capacity to restore homeostasis will depend on the number and severity of health events and life stressors, both past and present, as well as genetic predispositions.

Figure 2: The Path to Being Unwell

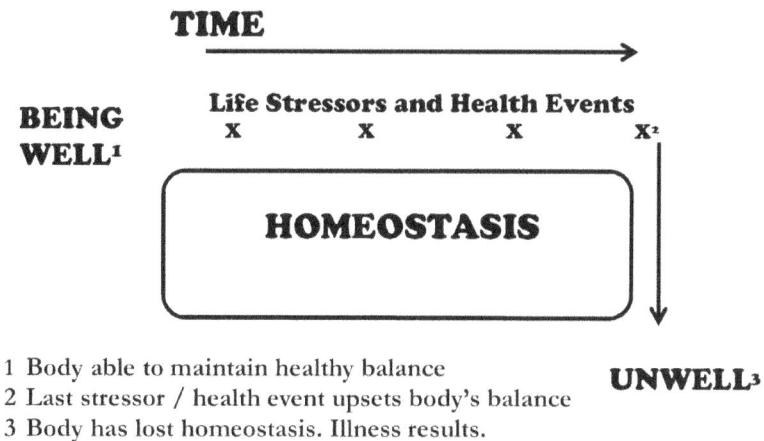

TIME

BEING WELL[1]

Life Stressors and Health Events

X   X   X   X[2]

HOMEOSTASIS

UNWELL[3]

1 Body able to maintain healthy balance
2 Last stressor / health event upsets body's balance
3 Body has lost homeostasis. Illness results.

Elements of Natural Healing

Restoring balance is reliant on natural healing, which involves several elements: a holistic assessment of function, dietary strategies, reducing toxic exposure, emotional balance, adequate rest, exercise, energy flow, nutritional supplements, restoring metabolic function, and addressing toxic accumulation (if present).

All natural healing begins with a **holistic assessment,** which helps determine the appropriate interventions. A holistic assessment involves taking a detailed history to identify life stressors and health events that may be involved in the loss of homeostasis. Important lines of inquiry include past illnesses (including those in childhood), emotionally trying experiences, toxic exposure, and past dietary habits. With my clients, I ask this revealing question: *Was there an event after which you never felt well again?* This typically reveals the point at which homeostasis was lost. An analysis of current symptoms and their severity will point to the specific body systems affected. This analysis, called *nutritional symptomatology*, is explained in Chapter 11. Holistic practitioners may use other tools in their assessment, such as applied kinesiology, iridology, live blood analysis, and galvanic skin response.

Dietary strategies vary according to the health issue. I use three strategies in succession to support natural healing:

A quality diet: Food is the foundation for natural healing. Too often, the role of food and nutrition is not addressed in mainstream medical treatment. Chapter 7 outlines my holistic definition of a quality diet.

Diet suited to individual needs: In Chapter 8, I offer the rationale for, and the process of, finding the diet that best supports being well. Eating the diet suited to our individual needs can help prevent illness, and, in my clinical experience, supports healing from many health conditions.

Healing diets: There are foods and liquids in specific combinations that can support or accelerate the natural healing process. Chapter 12 discusses how to use food for natural healing.

Toxic exposure must be reduced to allow the body to focus on healing work. Chapters 1 and 2 reveal evidence of several toxins in the food supply. Chapter 5 outlines the toxic threats from our physical environment.

Emotional balance, as discussed in Chapter 9, is a foundation for being well. Undue stress is a barrier to healing that I discuss in this chapter.

Adequate sleep is essential for all body systems—immune, digestion, hormones, circulation, respiration. Seven to eight hours of sleep nightly is typically required during the healing process.

Exercise has benefits that span the body and the mind. It can support healing but also hinder it. Ideally, exercise should be at a moderate level and intensity. Moderate physical movement supports healing through production of endorphins to boost mood, encouraging regular bowel elimination, and supporting the immune system. Exercise that is too strenuous or prolonged can interfere with the healing process. Exercise to build muscle or increase physical stamina is not the focus that will support natural healing.

To determine the exercise level that supports healing, the frequency, intensity, and duration of exercise must be considered. Moderate activity can mean as seldom as three times per week or as often as daily, depending on the duration and intensity. At three times per week, an hour of sustained movement provides great benefit, especially when it elevates the heart rate for at least 30 minutes. Daily exercise is also beneficial, but should be no more than 30-40 minutes of continuous activity, such as walking, biking, swimming, yoga, or dancing. Duration is determined by personal fitness level prior to starting a healing protocol. Intensity is similarly determined by your own fitness level. Taking the pulse periodically is the best way to keep your activity level from becoming too intense. A heart rate calculator can be found online at www.webmd.com. Choosing enjoyable activities is ideal; if exercise is not fun, we are less likely to do it.

Currently, I observe two exercise trends, neither of which is health supportive. Some people are exercising to excess, while others are "couch potatoes." During healing, too much exercise can be as damaging as too little. An attitude has taken hold in our society; if a little is good, a lot is better. Unfortunately, exercising too much can become a stressor that upsets the body's homeostasis. During strenuous exercise, free radicals form in the body that, if not neutralized, will attack healthy tissues and cells. A free radical is an unstable molecule that, in order to become stable, steals an electron and the only available source is from healthy body tissues. This action destabilizes and damages tissues, which can increase the risk of health problems. Those involved in strenuous pursuits—long-distance running, biking, contact sports—need to understand how to use micronutrients, such as antioxidants, to neutralize the harmful effects of free radicals. Chapter 13 provides information on antioxidants.

Energy flow through the body can be interrupted by illness and injury. Several energy therapies focus on opening the energy pathways that will promote healing. Effective energy therapies include Reiki, Bowen Therapy, Reflexology, Acupuncture, and Therapeutic Touch.

Restoring metabolic function is about optimizing three processes: digestion, absorption, and elimination. For healing to occur, food must be properly digested, nutrients absorbed, and waste eliminated. Chapter 11 discusses the symptoms of inefficient digestion, malabsorption, and poor elimination, and possible healing steps. Protocols to restore healthy balance to the digestive tract are outlined in Chapter 14.

Once homeostasis is lost, it may be difficult to restore healthy balance without taking one or more **nutritional supplements,** which may include vitamins, minerals, amino acids, enzymes, probiotics, essential fatty acids, herbs, glandular extracts, and homeopathic remedies. There are three ways to use supplements: therapeutic, supportive, and palliative. Only therapeutic and supportive use promotes natural healing.

Supplements become therapeutic when taken at an optimal dosage, frequency, and in a specific combination of micronutrients. This practice, termed orthomolecular nutrition, evolved from research by the famed Nobel laureate, Dr. Linus Pauling, who coined the term in 1968. The information website orthomolecularmedicine.com describes orthomolecular health as one that "aims to restore the optimum environment of the body by correcting imbalances or deficiencies based on individual biochemistry."[1] An orthomolecular approach can treat disease and mental illness, but in nutrition practice, the focus is on prevention through the therapeutic use of nutrients. Therapeutic-level supplements contain optimal micronutrient dosages and in combinations that work synergistically. Supplements containing therapeutic-level dosages are typically available only from holistic health practitioners (e.g., holistic nutritionists, naturopaths, and homeopaths). Such practitioners should also supervise the use of these supplements to ensure their intended benefit.

Supplements are supportive when they provide basic nutrients the body needs. For nutrient deficiencies resulting from illness or because of aging, I routinely recommend supportive supplements of vitamins, minerals, probiotics, and essential fatty acids, to name a few. A supportive product is typically at the dosage recommended by the manufacturer. Higher dosages represent therapeutic use.

A dictionary definition of the word palliative is to "relieve pain or alleviate a problem without dealing with the underlying cause." Taking supplements palliatively may make you feel better, but it does not promote natural healing, and often results in long-term reliance on the supplement. The complicated role of supplements in natural healing is covered in more detail in Chapter 13.

Toxic accumulation, if present, can be addressed with the application of a protocol called detoxification. The longer and more severe the imbalance, the more likely it is that toxins are involved. The process of detoxifying the body is discussed in Chapter 15.

Process of Natural Healing

Once a course of healing is identified, restoring homeostasis relies on taking steps in a specific order to honour the way our bodies naturally heal. The time needed for each step will depend on several factors: the degree of imbalance at the outset, compliance with the recommended dietary and lifestyle program, and the ability to control stress. The process that supports natural healing follows these steps:

1. Ensure your diet includes good quality foods
2. Determine the right diet for *you*
3. Follow a healing diet and use foods for healing
4. Use supplements therapeutically
5. Ensure efficient digestion, absorption, and elimination, e.g., cleansing
6. Detoxification, if needed

Emotional balance is not listed in these steps because it is a foundation for healing that may require ongoing attention. As outlined in Chapter 9, the search for emotional balance may be a lifelong quest. The next section deals with barriers to healing, one of which is an unhealthy response to stress.

Barriers to Healing

I routinely see two barriers to natural healing: chronic stress and over-reliance on medications to control symptoms.

Chronic Stress

The *busyness* of living in an industrialized society can leave many people chronically stressed. Unrelenting stress blocks the healing process through two body systems—hormonal and nervous. Hormones such as cortisol are released by the adrenal gland in response to events that we perceive as stressful. With continued and relentless stress, cortisol is continually in circulation. When cortisol is always active, sleep quality will always suffer. Cortisol levels normally decrease at night, so that we can relax and fall asleep. If you cannot get to sleep because your mind won't stop, elevated cortisol could be the culprit. In the long term, insomnia will weaken the body's functioning.

The nervous system is beautifully designed to deal with stress using two of its subsystems: the sympathetic and the parasympathetic. These systems are balanced so that when one is active, the other one is not. As discussed in Chapter 6, stress induces the sympathetic system to make us more alert and ready to act. This means that during emotional stress, the parasympathetic system is turned off. Since the parasympathetic system controls digestion, continual stress shuts down the digestive process. When we do not digest well, nutrient absorption is compromised and so, too, is our ability to heal. Even if the other elements of natural healing are addressed, undue stress will mean that progress is extremely slow, and, in some cases, healthy balance may never be restored.

Medications that control symptoms

The highest ideal of cure is the speedy, gentle, and enduring restoration of health by the most trustworthy and least harmful way. ~ Samuel Hahnemann, the founder of homeopathy

In the 21ˢᵗ century, there is a medication for almost everything, but drug therapies are a mixed blessing. There is value in some medications because people with serious ailments can carry on in ways not possible in the past. There is relief from chronic pain, high blood pressure, blood sugar imbalances, and anxiety. However, there are two problems with almost any medication, both prescribed and over-the-counter: they have side effects and they focus on symptom relief. In fact, side effects are a function of the mechanism by which most medications work. They target one protein that controls a body response related to an unwanted symptom. Unfortunately, the targeted protein has other functions that, while not the focus of the drug, are negatively affected. Harmful side effects often involve digestion, absorption, and elimination. Compromising these critical body functions will interfere with natural healing processes. I observe that, tragically, another medication may be prescribed to address the side effects of the first one.

Medications for acid reflux are a good example of symptom relief with side effects. The most common prescription antacid is the proton pump inhibitor (PPI) designed to block the production of stomach acid, thereby reducing acid reflux and indigestion. This has unfortunate ill effects because of the relationship between stomach acid and digestion. Stomach acid is needed to stimulate the release of digestive enzymes, and by blocking this process, digestion is impaired. This can result in poor absorption of nutrients, such as calcium, iron, magnesium, zinc, folic acid, and B vitamins. Warning signs of ill effects from PPIs include nausea, headache, bloating, and diarrhea—all signs of digestive malfunction. Other body systems can be affected as well. The *Family Health Guide* of Harvard Medical School links long-term use of PPIs to pneumonia, *Clostridium difficile* (C. difficile) infection, and increased risk of osteoporosis and bone fractures.[2]

The following are commonly used medications and their associated potential side effects that interfere with healing:

Antidepressants: Slow down the metabolism, causing constipation and tendency to gain weight

Antibiotics: Destroy all bacteria in the body, both harmful and beneficial. We need beneficial bacteria in the gut to aid in digestion and absorption of nutrients. Poorly nourished bodies are prone to illness. Overuse of antibiotics has also triggered the development of antibiotic-resistant bacteria, a serious risk to health.

Antihistamines: Encourage water excretion, which can increase risk of dehydration. Poor hydration interferes with healing. Other side effects include loss of appetite, nausea, upset stomach, dizziness, and drowsiness.

Salicylates (e.g., *Aspirin*): Wear down the lining of the stomach, which may trigger ulcers and stomach bleeding. Digestion is adversely affected, which also reduces absorption of nutrients. Eventually, immune deficiencies can result.

Analgesics (i.e., ibuprofen, acetaminophen): One common use is to lower fevers, a natural immune defense that serves an important purpose in fighting infections. Viruses cannot survive at high temperatures, which is why the human immune system mounts a fever in response. If a mild-to-moderate fever is lowered with medication, natural healing can be suppressed. In his book *Never Be Sick Again*, Raymond Francis refers to several studies in the 1990s showing that long-term use of analgesics was linked to ulcers, kidney failure, cognitive dysfunction, hearing loss, and hormone disruption.[3]

In 2000, a report in the *Journal of the American Medical Association* questioned the medical system's reliance on prescription drugs. Two issues were raised. Based on its level of spending on health care, Americans' health status should be better than it is. Worse still, an estimated 100,000 people die from medical errors, of which many are because of adverse reactions to medications.[4]

By providing symptom relief, medications can also stop the search for root causes of health concerns. Without symptoms to warn us, our body function could deteriorate unnoticed until other health issues arise. For this reason, I view medications taken for symptom relief as a serious barrier to the healing process. If medications are considered medically essential, their side effects may be addressed with the help of a holistic health practitioner.

The Experience of Natural Healing

The time required to heal naturally is a function of several factors, including the time spent being unwell, the health issue in question, and the severity of symptoms. Homeostasis might be restored in a few months, but it could also take a few years. In addition, natural healing is not a linear process proceeding directly from illness to wellness. Variable progress in healing can be accompanied by symptoms that, in holistic health practice, are known as the *healing crisis* or *healing reaction*.

In a natural healing protocol, the body is working to restore healthy balance and, during a protocol, there may be toxins released that create unpleasant symptoms. Healing reactions often occur in the initial stages of a protocol, but also when the body makes a significant breakthrough. Rapid changes from a poor diet to a healthier one can be enough to cause discomfort.

While healing reactions may be unpleasant, they are signs that healing is occurring. Healing reactions vary from person to person and can include headaches; fever and/or colds; skin rashes/eruptions; a short interval of bowel sluggishness; occasional diarrhea; tiredness and weakness; nervousness; irritability; negativity or depression; and frequent urination. There is often the temptation to take medications (e.g., pain relievers) to ease healing reactions, but this can interfere with the healing process. I always alert my clients to the possibility of a healing reaction, so they do not mistake it as an illness. Those who have enjoyed the benefits of natural healing persisted through these apparent setbacks. Symptoms should be short-lived and tolerable, but if they persist, this points to a more serious condition that should be assessed by a medical doctor.

Supporting the Body's Healing Processes

Several health habits and choices support the natural healing process:

- Drink at least one quart of filtered water per 100 pounds of body weight per day. This helps flush out toxins and helps cleanse the kidneys. Acceptable filtration methods and other fluid sources are discussed in Chapter 7.
- Increase intake of fruits, vegetables, bran from oats (wheat bran is often too scratchy and irritating), and high-fibre foods, such as ground flax or chia seed. These steps help accelerate toxin removal and keep bowels moving.
- Keep active on a daily basis. Walking for fifteen minutes is often enough. Mild exercise supports the body's detoxification processes.
- For the first two weeks of any healing protocol, sleep at least eight hours each night.
- Avoid medications that could slow the healing process.
- Seek guidance from a health care professional who can properly interpret symptoms and healing reactions.

Natural healing is about honouring how the body works to restore health, which is not negotiable—the body works the way it works and cannot be sidestepped or fooled. Unfortunately, our desire for a speedy recovery can tempt us to bypass natural healing processes. Such attempts, even taking an analgesic for a headache, can block or delay healing. Supporting the body's return to homeostasis involves some required elements that need to be followed in a specific order. Those who will stay the course can return from almost any imbalance.

Before natural healing can begin, we must assess where body function is out of balance, and in holistic nutrition, this is effectively done through analysis of bodily symptoms. In the next chapter, I discuss what body symptoms mean and how they are used to select the appropriate healing protocols.

Chapter Notes

1. *Orthomolecular Medicine, Orthomed.org,* accessed August 12, 2014, http://www.orthomed.org/.

2. "Do PPI's have long term side effects?" *Harvard Medical School, Family Health Guide, Online Companion,* accessed August 12, 2014, http://www.health.harvard.edu/fhg/updates/do-ppis-have-long-term-side-effects.shtml.

3. Raymond Francis, MSc, *Never Be Sick Again: Health Is a Choice, Learn How to Choose It* (Deerfield Beach, Florida: Health Communications, Inc., 2002), 299.

4. Barbara Starfield, MD, "Is U.S. Health Really the Best in the World?" *Journal of the American Medical Association* 284 no.4 (2000): 483-485, accessed August 14, 2014, doi:10.1001/jama.284.4.483.

11: LISTEN TO YOUR BODY

Be aware of the importance of addressing interactive factors, which are unique to each individual. ~ Guiding Principle of Holistic Nutrition, Canadian School of Natural Nutrition

The body speaks to us in the language of symptoms which, when properly understood, tell a detailed story about our body's functioning. This clinical knowledge is called *nutritional symptomatology* and is different in focus to *symptomatology*—the medical science of symptoms or the combined symptoms of a disease. Nutritional symptomatology is an analysis of symptom patterns that reflect how the body is functioning, rather than indicators of illness. Poor function always precedes illness, so, by detecting functional problems and taking action to address them, illness may be prevented or identified sooner. Nutritional symptomatology is the primary assessment tool used by holistic nutritionists to assess body function and determine healing interventions.

Bodily symptoms tell us when there is malfunction and can guide us to appropriate healing steps. Take, for example, symptoms that you no doubt understand. If you sprain your ankle, there is sudden pain and swelling. If you keep walking on the ankle, healing will not occur. However, you are more likely to respond to the pain by resting the ankle and perhaps using ice to reduce the swelling. Here, symptoms (pain and swelling) will point to healing steps (rest and ice). Not all symptoms are this easy to understand, and act on. Some are warning signs of an illness that must be assessed by a medical doctor before turning to nutritional symptomatology. For example, a severe headache and stiff neck can be a sign of serious illness, such as polio or meningitis. When there is no medically diagnosed illness, nutritional symptomatology is an effective tool to investigate functional health issues.

Considered separately, each symptom may not tell us what is going on. Nutritional symptomatology considers bodily symptoms in combinations or patterns. Also important are symptom onset, severity, and their relationship to health history and life events. Understanding and analyzing all this information is the strength of holistic nutrition practice. Before explaining nutritional symptomatology, it is important to distinguish it from the medical consideration of symptoms.

Medical Consideration of Symptoms

Long before there were medical tests, doctors used symptoms as the primary assessment tool for diagnosing illness. Today, doctors rely heavily on tests—blood work, X-rays, computerized topography (CT scans), ultrasounds, electroencephalography (EEGs), electrocardiogram (EKGs), magnetic resonance imaging (MRIs)—to the point of believing test results over the patients' symptoms. My personal experience with this was most distressing:

> I vividly recall when the gastroenterologist told me that my daughter, then 14 years old, was "basically healthy." He had completed all the tests at his disposal and, finding nothing, reached this conclusion. At that point, my daughter has been suffering for two and a half years with nausea, fatigue, and loss of mental acuity, which severely reduced her ability to function. She missed so much school, she was failing her courses and did not have energy for any kind of social life. Faced with her continuing debilitating symptoms, the doctor chose instead to believe his test results. (I have since heard this complaint from many of my clients whose doctors told them there was nothing wrong with them). Thankfully, I chose not to believe the specialist's "basically healthy" pronouncement. I found an alternative health practitioner who focused on interpreting her symptoms and health history and the protocol that led to my daughter's eventual return to health.

Medical doctors do not always ignore symptoms. Sometimes when they cannot explain symptoms, they put a disease label on them. I believe this is why there are new "diseases", such as gastro-esophageal reflux disease (GERD), irritable bowel syndrome (IBS), chronic fatigue syndrome (CFS), and asthma. I call these *symptom-conditions* because they are more a set of symptoms than an assessment of causes. Unfortunately, having such diagnoses can stop the search for underlying causes, because all the focus is on the symptoms, and relieving them. It is no coincidence that there are prescription medications and over-the-counter drugs to address these symptom-conditions. For these four conditions, the medical and holistic health approaches are very different.

Gastro-Esophageal Reflux Disease (GERD)

This condition has two main symptoms: acid reflux and burning in the stomach. The medical view is that GERD is caused by excess stomach acid. Ironically, the holistic health view is that low stomach acid is often the underlying issue. It may seem odd that acid reflux stems from low stomach acid. Naturopath and author, Dr. John Matsen, explains how stomach acid acts as a natural antibiotic to control microbes that can grow in the stomach. If stomach acid is low, these microbes can grow, ferment, and even putrefy food in the stomach often resulting in excess gas, acid reflux and heartburn.[1]

Another medical explanation for GERD is the malfunction of the sphincter at the entrance of the stomach (also known as a hiatal hernia). What is causing the malfunction? Matsen considers hiatal hernias to result from long-term poor diet (e.g., SAD) and/or stress, which cause the esophagus to spasm, allowing stomach acid to splash up into the esophagus.[2] The root cause of GERD in either case is not high stomach acid, yet the standard medical treatment is to reduce acid with medication.

Taking antacids for GERD inhibits digestion, in particular of proteins, and over time, malnutrition can develop. This can manifest in several ways and did so most dramatically with one of my clients.

J.K., aged 75, came to me with persistent reflux. She could not get through the day without several naps, was unsteady on her feet, and could not drive her car because she had blacked out several times. She had been taking a prescription antacid for five years, with little relief in her symptoms. After I recommended she change her diet to eliminate sensitive foods, her GERD symptoms were relieved, her energy returned, and she no longer needed to take an antacid medication. In the process of regaining health, she also required nutritional supplements because of prolonged nutrient deficits.

To summarize, the underlying causes for GERD symptoms stem from one or more of these factors: poor diet, food sensitivities, undue stress, lingering bacterial infections (e.g., Helicobacter pylori), lingering viral infections, parasitic infections, sluggish metabolism, and accumulation of toxins. All these issues respond to holistic nutrition protocols.

Irritable Bowel Syndrome (IBS)

IBS is the most common condition among my clients and, sadly, most report that their medical doctor gave them little hope of relief. Some were taking prescribed anti-inflammatory medications, but then experienced side effects, such as constipation and weight gain. A 2012 study investigated psychological and group therapy as a treatment for IBS, with mixed results—only those with the lowest quality of life found some relief. The researchers state, "The exact causes [of IBS] are not well understood."[3] The holistic health view is that the *irritation* of the digestive tract is due to one or more of these factors: poor-quality diet; wrong diet for individual needs; food intolerances, physical damage to the intestinal villi from past poor diet or parasites; side effects of medication (antibiotics, antidepressants, antihistamines); and issues with handling stress. The IBS symptoms of abdominal bloating and pain represent poor function of the bowels and perhaps also the liver and pancreas. My clients report considerable relief in their IBS symptoms with diet change alone once they know which foods are irritating to them. Protocols to address IBS may include: healing diets, cleansing, detoxification, and stress management (counseling, spiritual discovery, meditation, Reiki, yoga, tai chi).

Chronic Fatigue Syndrome (CFS)

Chronic fatigue is a relatively new condition and primarily seen in the industrialized western world. Diagnosis of CFS is unusual because it is established by first excluding other causes. The educational website Medicine.net defines chronic fatigue syndrome as "severe chronic fatigue of six months or longer duration with other known medical conditions excluded. Four or more of the following symptoms are present: substantial impairment in short-term memory or concentration; sore throat; tender lymph nodes; muscle pain; multi-joint pain without swelling or redness; headaches of a new type, pattern or severity; non-refreshing sleep; and post-exertion malaise lasting over 24 hours."[4]

There is no medical cure for CFS, but symptoms may be controlled with prescription pain medication. Naturopath and alternative health educator, Lilieana Stadler Mitrea, identifies several issues that could underly CFS: "Persistent viral infections; stress/low adrenal function; weak/non-optimal immune system; pre-existing physical conditions (cardio-vascular disease, multiple sclerosis, diabetes, cancer, etc.); depression; or impaired liver function."[5] Anything that challenges the immune system—toxic overload, the wrong diet, parasites—can be involved, but I have observed that an unhealthy response to stress often plays a role. In my clinical practice, therapeutic protocols are usually required to make any difference in symptoms of CFS. However, diet change is seldom enough; restoring emotional balance is also critical, as discussed in Chapter 9.

Asthma

While the incidence of asthma has risen dramatically in North America, the Asthma Society of Canada states on its website "the cause of asthma is not known."[6] In *Allergies: Disease in Disguise*, naturopath Carolee Bateson-Koch maintains that asthma is associated with one or more factors: food sensitivities, diet high in damaged fat, chronic infection (bacteria, virus, parasites), and digestive enzyme deficiency.[7] My clinical experience supports these asthma links. The most common presenting issue I find among clients living with asthma is sensitivity to one or more foods such as dairy, wheat, and/or soy. Additives associated with asthma include sulphites, used as a food preservative, the food dye Yellow Dye #5 (Tartrazine), and the flavouring agent monosodium glutamate. Processed foods with these additives also typically contain trans fats and/or damaged fats, which promote inflammation in the body. When my clients eliminate their sensitive foods and stop eating foods that contain additives and damaged fats, they invariably have fewer asthma symptoms. It is interesting to note that the dramatic increase in asthma in North America has coincided with the introduction of processed foods.

An imbalance in the intestinal tract can also underlie asthma. This imbalance, termed dysbiosis, can involve an overgrowth of mold/fungus and/or parasites. Various parasites live in the intestines and the damage they cause impairs the ability to digest and absorb nutrients. Dysfunction of one elimination pathway (intestines), whether from mold/fungus or parasites, negatively affects another pathway, in this case, the lungs. Many of my clients who suffer from asthma turn out to have long-term parasitic infections. Their asthma medication (e.g., puffers) provides symptom relief, but does not get to the root of the problem—a dysbiosis. Chapter 14 explains these digestive imbalances and the appropriate holistic nutrition interventions.

I find it tragic that the medical solution for these four symptom-conditions is medication that focuses on symptom relief only. These are not healing solutions because the medications are needed indefinitely and they have side effects (see Chapter 10) that will interfere with natural healing. However, a holistic nutrition approach can address the root causes through diet and lifestyle changes and sometimes time-limited therapeutic protocols. In the next section, I explain how to use nutritional symptomatology to identify poor body function *before* it develops into illness.

Prevention through Nutritional Symptomatology

Nutritional symptomatology is an extremely valuable tool for the prevention of serious or chronic illness. Symptoms point to poor bodily function, which always precedes illness and often by several years. For example, type 2 diabetes is a malfunction in managing glucose and balancing blood sugar. Before a diagnosis of diabetes, there are symptoms such as cravings for sweets, unusual thirst, being hungry soon after eating, and irritability from missing a meal. Nutritional symptomatology sees these as the early signs of diabetes, which may be prevented by making timely dietary changes. Blood sugar imbalances can go on for years before physical illness or disease develops—plenty of time to take preventative action.

Nutritional symptomatology, with considerable accuracy, pinpoints how the body is malfunctioning. There are dozens of symptom patterns I use as assessment tools, but five symptom patterns are the most telling indicators of poor health function that can lead to illness: stomach function, underactive; stomach function, overactive; liver/gall bladder stress; kidney/bladder stress; and intestinal imbalance. Known in the holistic nutrition field, these malfunctions are the most common ones I see in clinical practice. For each symptom pattern, I offer my supportive steps in an approximate order to be investigated. If symptoms are relieved after the first few steps, the remaining ones are unnecessary. Some steps are marked with an asterisk because these interventions require consultation with a health practitioner, either mainstream medical or holistic.

NOTE: To address the symptom patterns below, there are five foundational steps—quality diet, a diet right for individual needs, toxin-free environment, ruling out food and/or chemical sensitivities, and emotional balance. These five foundations are covered in Part 2: Holistic Guides to Being Well. Consider these foundational steps as required prerequisites to the supportive steps offered here.

Stomach Function, underactive

This malfunction occurs when the stomach is not producing enough hydrochloric acid or digestive enzymes to process food. In my clinical practice, I have observed it is not necessary to have all the following symptoms for this functional issue to exist. Common symptoms of an underactive stomach include:

Excessive gas, belching, or burping after eating

Feel tired after eating

Heavy feeling in the stomach after eating

Abdominal bloating

Longitudinal lines or ridges on fingernails (indicates a long-term issue)

Supportive Steps for Underactive stomach (*may require consultation with a health-care practitioner):

- Eat slowly and chew food well. This activates enzymes in the saliva and stomach
- Avoid washing meals down with fluids, which dilutes digestive juices
- Follow the Digestive Balancing diet—*See Chapter 12*
- Rule out bacterial infections, such as Helicobacter pylori*--*See Chapter 14*
- Rule out sluggish metabolism, caused by long-term low-calorie diets or low thyroid function

Stomach Function, overactive

This issue is typically identified as high acidity in the stomach. Common symptoms include:

> Stomach pain after eating
> Burning sensation in stomach
> Heartburn, indigestion not related to any food
> Stomach pain aggravated by emotional stress
> Nausea

Notice that symptoms of underactive and overactive stomach are similar, which can make it difficult to determine which one is the issue. Holistic nutritionist Danielle Perrault offers this simple self-test for hyperacidity: "…when pain or discomfort (heartburn) is experienced 40 to 60 minutes after a meal and is quickly relieved by taking an antacid."[8]

Supportive Steps for Overactive Stomach (*may require consultation with health practitioner):

- Avoid spicy and fried foods
- Avoid taking aspirin, which further irritates the stomach
- Avoid processed foods and foods low in fibre—*See Chapter 7*
- Use healing foods. Have soothers and avoid stimulants such as caffeine—*See Chapter 12*
- Rule out a hiatal hernia or ulcer*

With my clientele, the more common imbalance is an underactive stomach. Identifying whether the stomach is under- or overactive often requires consultation with a holistic nutritionist.

Liver/Gall bladder Stress

The liver is the powerhouse of the body because it has over 100 functions involving circulation, excretion, metabolism, detoxification, bile production, and hormone regulation. Compromise of any of these functions, upsets homeostasis and results in ill health. Gall bladder function is closely associated with liver health.

Because of the liver's numerous vital functions (about 500), symptoms of liver/gall bladder stress are varied. Common symptoms of liver (and possibly gall bladder) stress are:

Bad breath or bad taste in mouth

Oily skin around nose, or on forehead

Constipation

Stool is yellow in colour

Acne, boils, rashes, eczema

Weight gain in the abdominal area

Migraine headaches

With at least three symptoms present, I would suspect poor function of the liver and/or gall bladder.

Supportive Steps for Liver/Gall bladder Stress (*may require consultation with a health practitioner):

- Limit intake of alcohol, which challenges the liver's detoxification functions
- Eat supportive foods, such as beets (leaf and root) and dandelion greens; add fresh lemon juice to your drinking water
- Eat only enough calories to meet needs and, if needed, lose weight
- If taking medications, check for side effects relating to symptoms of liver stress*--*See Chapter 10*
- Use the Digestive Balancing diet and avoid stimulants—*See Chapter 12*
- Ensure metabolism of fat is working efficiently
- Cleanse bowels*--*See Chapter 14*
- Rule out accumulation of toxins*--*See Chapter 15*

Kidney/Bladder Stress

The kidneys are the final filter of waste in liquid form. When there are too many waste products to filter, the kidney and/or the bladder (the holding area for waste fluids) will become irritated. Typically, when this happens, detoxification in the liver may also be incomplete. For this reason, stress to the kidneys can also point to poor liver function. Many of my clients suffer from symptoms of both imbalances that point to a more serious state. Common symptoms of kidney/bladder stress include:

Puffy under the eyes

Urgent and/or frequent urination

Low back pain

Tendency to urinary tract infections

Joint pains

Supportive Steps for Kidneys/Bladder Stress (*may require consultation with a health practitioner):

- Avoid caffeine, which is dehydrating—*See Chapter 12*

- If taking prescription medications, check to see if these symptoms are a side effect
- Use the Digestive balancing diet—*See Chapter 12*
- Cleanse bowels*--*See Chapter 14*
- Rule out accumulation of toxins*--*See Chapter 15*

Intestinal Imbalance

The small and large bowels handle the final stages of digestion, absorption of nutrients, and elimination of solid waste. The small bowel is the site of nutrient processing whereby enzymes break food down into small-enough particles to be absorbed. The large bowel contains microorganisms, both beneficial and pathogenic, that are needed in the right balance for bowel health and assimilation of nutrients, such as vitamin B12, iron, and vitamin K. Deficiency of these nutrients is almost always associated with an unhealthy balance in the intestines. Common symptoms of intestinal imbalance are:

Fatigue
Constipation and/or irregularity
Loose stools, chronic
Uncomfortable bowel movements
Abdominal gas and bloating
Mucous in stools
Flatulence
Hemorrhoids

Supportive Steps for Intestinal Imbalance (*may require consultation with health practitioner):

- Avoid overuse of antibiotics, which can upset bacterial balance
- Use healing foods: Anti-inflammatory diet; fermented foods; soothers—*See Chapter 12*
- Cleanse bowels*–*See Chapter 14*
- Rule out accumulation of toxins*–*See Chapter 15*
- Females: If using oral contraceptives over 5 years, consider alternatives

I would stress that the supportive steps for these five symptom patterns may not all be required. If symptoms are relieved by applying dietary changes—always the first step—then more therapeutic steps may not be needed.

Factors in Symptom Analysis

An in-depth analysis of symptoms is the key to identifying the ideal healing protocol. The importance of symptoms depends on three factors: duration, frequency, and timing. Duration and age of onset reveal the level of severity. Long-term issues of several years' duration are more serious and more likely call for therapeutic protocols. Daily incidence is more apt to indicate a malfunction in digestion, absorption, and elimination. Weekly symptoms must be considered in the context of lifestyle and diet and how they vary over the week. The time of day is also important; symptoms in the morning, afternoon, and evening can all mean something different. In general, morning symptoms after a full night of sleep can point to a more serious issue, while evening issues can be because of natural fatigue from the day or food that is consumed regularly. A thorough holistic assessment also includes health history, physical environment, and emotional balance.

SELF-HELP TIP: Keep a detailed daily journal of foods and fluids consumed, as well as any symptoms experienced during the day. This allows you to listen to your body and use that information to make health-promoting changes.

Common Symptoms and Their Nutritional Links

In the previous section, I showed how nutritional symptomatology analyzes multiple symptoms that occur in defined patterns. It is also helpful to understand individual symptoms, in particular common ones, that may relate to several possible nutritional imbalances. I observe many people put up with some common concerns—fatigue, headaches, nasal congestion, and skin rashes—because they cannot pinpoint the cause(s). Often, nutritional links are not even considered. These issues can all be relieved by over-the-counter products (e.g., energy drinks, painkillers, antihistamines, and skin creams), but these products mask the symptoms rather than addressing the underlying cause(s). In the absence of an illness (viral or bacterial infection, etc.) or physical injury, these symptoms are often related to dietary choices or a malfunction in a body response that a holistic nutrition protocol can address.

Fatigue is normal after hard work, exercise, or an illness. Unexplained fatigue is of more concern. When you wake up tired or have an energy dip in mid-afternoon, it is a sign of a bodily imbalance. In the absence of illness, holistic health practitioners view fatigue as a reflection of poor body function, of which there are several possibilities:

Nutritional deficiency

A poor-quality diet lacks vital nutrients. The body will not get enough vitamins and minerals to be properly supported. Fatigue is more common after long term adherence to a poor-quality diet.

Malabsorption of nutrients

The body is not absorbing nutrients well. Check for symptoms of underactive stomach, liver stress, or intestinal imbalance. Nutrient absorption can be restored with diet and supplements that support digestion. Ideally, this should be done under the direction of a holistic health practitioner.

Sluggish metabolism

Hypothyroidism—underactive thyroid—slows down the metabolism and can produce fatigue. Clients who come to me with sluggish metabolisms often have a history of severe calorie-restricted diets or gaining and losing weight repeatedly, often referred to as yo-yo dieting. With each successive weight loss, the metabolic rate is slowed further, and this makes it more difficult to maintain a healthy weight. There are dietary steps to stimulate the metabolism: eat nutrient-dense foods, eat small amounts frequently, and exercise regularly. Eating healthy fats also boosts the metabolic rate.

Sensitivity

Fatigue often follows consumption of a food or food additive to which you are sensitive. This can happen within a few hours or be delayed until the next day. My clients who eliminate foods to which they are sensitive almost always experience increased energy.

Toxicity from chemicals/heavy metals

Gradually worsening fatigue over several years can be a symptom of toxic accumulation in the body. Two factors point to toxic overload: exposure to toxins and the body's ability to eliminate them. Mainstream medical testing is not focused on assessing toxic accumulation unless there is known exposure to a chemical or heavy metal. Consulting with a holistic health practitioner will determine if toxicity is an issue (see Chapter 15).

Headaches often accompany illness from a virus or bacterial infection, but can also result from fatigue, hunger, excess sun exposure, whiplash, changes in barometric pressure, emotional stress, and hangovers. For women, pre-menses can trigger headaches. Nutritional symptomatology provides more clues to headache triggers, as follows:

Food sensitivity

Some foods that are commonly considered healthy can, in some people, produce headaches. When an individual is intolerant to one or more foods, there are several possible symptoms, one of which is a headache.

Food additives

Certain food additives can trigger headaches, e.g., MSG, aspartame, food dyes. Tip: Eat a diet free of these additives for a month. If headaches are reduced, suspect the culprit to be one or more additives.

Deficiency of vitamin B5

This vitamin, often referred to as the "anti-stress" vitamin, is not easily depleted because B5 is contained in so many foods (beef, eggs, fresh vegetables, organ meats, legumes, nuts, pork, saltwater fish, and whole grains). However, chronic stress can lead to a deficiency. Supplementation with B5 may be required.

Making dietary improvements

Ironically, changing from poor- to good-quality foods can produce headaches, at least initially, as a healing reaction. The worse the old diet was, the more likelihood of headaches while switching to a healthier way of eating. This is attributed to the body's release of toxins accumulated from a poor diet. Abruptly eliminating sugar and coffee after a period of excess consumption will typically produce headaches.

Even if you have only one coffee daily, this may occur. This is one symptom of a healing crisis or healing reaction, which is explained in Chapter 10, in the section, The Experience of Natural Healing.

Detoxification response

Headaches are common while undergoing a detoxification protocol. Dr. John Matsen explains this arises because toxins are being released beyond the body's ability to handle.[9] I see this most often in the initial days of detoxification. This is explained further in Chapter 15.

Medications

The information website Drugs.com reports headaches as potential side effects of several medications, including some of the most commonly prescribed, such as cholesterol-lowering (e.g., *Lipitor, Crestor*); antidepressants *(e.g., Paxil, Wellbutrin, Zoloft)*; blood sugar control (e.g., *Metformin*); sedatives (e.g., *Ambien*); and cardiovascular drugs, in particular ACE inhibitors (e.g., *Lisinopril).*[10]

Nasal congestion may accompany a cold or virus and allergies (seasonal, environmental, pets), but may also relate to the following nutritional and functional issues:

Certain foods

Dairy products are mucous forming. Congestion from allergies or a head cold can be made worse by consuming dairy products.

Food sensitivity

Any food sensitivity can manifest as nasal congestion. I suffered with this for years before I identified my dairy intolerance. Clinically, I observe congestion in connection with sensitivities to wheat and corn (See Chapter 8).

Toxic overload

The accumulation of chemicals in the body (pesticides, inhaled fumes, heavy metals) challenges the immune system. One immune response is to produce mucous in the nasal cavity.

Medications

Drugs.com lists stuffy nose as a potential side effect of the following prescription drugs: antidepressants (e.g., *Celexa or Cymbalta*); cholesterol lowering (e.g., *Lipitor*); sedatives (e.g., *Ambien*).[11]

Skin rashes are sometimes present with viral infections and fevers. Otherwise, rashes have their roots in diet and various functional issues:

Sensitivity

Eczema is a common condition associated with unidentified sensitivities to foods, additives or chemicals.

Chemical sensitivities

Chemicals in personal care products can irritate the skin. One such chemical is sodium lauryl sulfate found in body wash, shampoo, and laundry detergent.

Overgrowth of mold and fungus

An overgrowth of mold and fungus can move from the intestinal tract to a system-wide imbalance, which can affect other body systems, such as the skin.

Additives

The artificial sweetener aspartame can cause several symptoms, one of which is a skin rash.

Medications

Drugs.com reports rashes as potential side effects of antidepressants and cholesterol-lowering medications.[12] However, a rash can result from any medication that the liver cannot eliminate from circulation after the drug's function is completed. There is a greater likelihood of a rash side effect in the presence of liver stress, a health imbalance discussed earlier in this chapter.

In summary, the key points about listening to your body's symptoms are:

- If a medical evaluation rules out illness and disease, continue searching for answers in poor bodily functions.
- Malfunction will always precede illness, often for several years. But malfunction will be accompanied by symptoms, which serve as early warning signs that should not be ignored.
- Avoid medicating symptoms until the cause(s) of illness or malfunction are known.
- Nutritional symptomatology can direct healing protocols that restore healthy function.
- Five symptom patterns underlie many health conditions: underactive stomach, overactive stomach, liver/gall bladder stress, kidney/bladder stress, and intestinal imbalance. For each symptom pattern, there are several supportive steps to help determine their cause(s); however, if there are multiple issues, you may require the help of a holistic nutritionist.
- Some common symptoms are indicators of functional imbalances for which there are natural healing solutions available only from a holistic health perspective. Avoid medicating these symptoms away before seeking their underlying cause(s).

Chapter Notes

1. John Matsen, ND, *Eating Alive: Prevention thru Good Digestion* (North Vancouver, British Columbia: Compton Books, 2002), 11.

2. Ibid., 5-8.

3. United States, Department of Health and Human Services, National Institute of Diabetes, Digestive and Kidney Diseases, "Brief Psychological and Educational Therapy Improves Symptoms of Irritable Bowel Syndrome" (December 3, 2012), accessed March 10, 2014, http://www.niddk.nih.gov/news/research-updates/Pages/brief-psychological-educational-therapy-improves-symptoms-irritable-bowel-syndrome.aspx.

4. "What are the signs and symptoms of chronic fatigue syndrome?" *medicinenet.com,* (July 3, 2013), accessed March 10, 2014, http://www.medicinenet.com/chronic_fatigue_syndrome/page4.htm#what_are_the_symptoms_and_signs_of_chronic_fatigue_syndrome.

5. Lilieana Stadler Mitrea, MD (Eur), ND, DNM, *Pathology and Nutrition: A Guide for Professionals,* First edition revised (Richmond Hill, Ontario: CSNN Publishing, a division of the Canadian School of Natural Nutrition, 2005), 257.

6. "Asthma Facts and Statistics," *Asthma Society of Canada, asthma.ca,* accessed August 12, 2014, http://www.asthma.ca/adults/about/asthma_facts_and_statistics.pdf.

7. Carolee Bateson-Koch, DC, ND, *Allergies: Disease in Disguise* (Burnaby, British Columbia: Alive Books, 1994), 126, 199.

8. Danielle Perrault, RHN, *Nutritional Symptomatology* (Richmond Hill, Ontario: CSNN Publishing, a division of the Canadian School of Natural Nutrition, 2000), 26.

9. John Matsen, ND, *Eating Alive: Prevention thru Good Digestion* (North Vancouver, British Columbia: Compton Books, 2002).

10. "Drug side effects," *drugs.com,* accessed August 15, 2014, http://www.drugs.com/sfx/.

11. Ibid.

12. Ibid.

12: USE FOOD FOR HEALING

Let your food be your medicine and your medicine be your food. ~ Ancient Greek philosopher Hippocrates, considered the "father of modern medicine"

Ancient wisdom held that food is integral to healing. Unfortunately, today's medical practice has little to do with food. A doctor might recommend that you *eat better*, but is unlikely to offer specific suggestions or include diet in his or her treatment plan. If you have been in hospital and eaten the meals there, you know they are not trying to heal you through nutrition.

Of course, Hippocrates is correct. Our food choices can support healing from illness and disease. I have clients who experienced healing in relation to acid reflux, allergies, anxiety, attention deficit disorder, high blood pressure, blood sugar imbalance, Crohn's, headaches, irritable bowel syndrome, rashes, premenstrual syndrome, and menopausal problems all by changing what/how/when they ate. Prior to my diet protocols, most of these clients had been resigned to suffering from these conditions. Many took prescription medications to get through each day and endured their side effects. I helped them discover that foods, food combinations, eating patterns, and preparation methods all enhance the body's recuperative powers.

I use several dietary protocols that support natural healing for a wide range of health issues. For each protocol, I outline how they are beneficial and which issue(s) they address. I start with approaches that are generally beneficial and conclude with those that apply to specific health conditions.

Digestive Balancing

This basic healing protocol is supportive as a starting point for most people. I recommend it for those who have no serious illness but suffer from one or more of the symptom patterns discussed in Chapter 11—Stomach function, underactive or overactive; liver/gall bladder stress; kidney/bladder stress; and intestinal imbalance. I also recommend this protocol as a trial diet to help identify food sensitivities (see Chapter 8). The "Foods to Have" are easy to digest and contain health-promoting nutrients. The "Foods to Avoid" are more difficult to digest or contain additives or substances (hormones, antibiotics) that impair healthy function of several body systems. This diet can be followed for extended periods of time (see Appendix 2).

Food Combining

Using Digestive Balancing as the diet foundation, there are ways to combine foods for healing, specifically for those with low levels of digestive enzymes (see Chapter 11 "Stomach function, underactive"). Because the main food groups—proteins, carbohydrates, and fats—are digested at different rates, there are ways to combine foods that reduces stress on the digestive process. Carbohydrates comprising simple sugars (simple carbs) digest the fastest, while proteins digest the slowest. For some people, eating simple carbs and proteins at the same time can lead to digestive upsets. Slow-burning proteins are apt to block the proper digestion of the fast-burning carbs, which ferment in the stomach, resulting in indigestion, reflux, or gas. The practice of combining foods that digest at the same or a similar rate is a widely accepted nutrition intervention, as follows:

Ideal Food Combining

High-protein and non-starch vegetables, e.g., chicken and salad

High-starch and non-starch vegetables, e.g., potatoes and broccoli

Healthy oils and most vegetables, e.g., salad and oil-based dressing

- Best sources of healthy oils include ocean fish, flax, pumpkin, sesame, safflower, and sunflower oils and their seeds.

Good Food Combining

High-starch and healthy oils, e.g., pasta with olive oil

Poor Food Combining

High-protein and high-starch (i.e., steak and potato or corn; a hamburger)

High-protein and fruit*—especially eating fruit after a meat-based meal

High-starch and fruit, e.g., fruit eaten after a pasta-based meal; fruit pie

*The ideal is to eat fruit one hour before or two to three hours after a meal

For those who suffer from chronic ailments, "ideal" or "good" food combining is recommended ongoing. For others, this may be a temporary healing protocol after an acute illness or cancer treatments. Radiation of the abdomen and chemotherapy treatments impairs intestinal function, which upsets digestion and nutrient absorption.

Alkaline Balancing

Our capacity to heal is highly related to the body's acid-alkaline balance. Over-acidity is not about levels of stomach acid; it is about system-wide acid/alkaline imbalances. In her book *The Body Ecology Diet: Recovering Your Health and Rebuilding Your Immunity*, Donna Gates warns that prolonged over-acidity in the body will make us more susceptible to illness from bacteria, viruses, and parasites, resulting in symptoms such as persistent fatigue, arthritis, and allergies.[1] It is also widely accepted that cancer cells thrive in an acidic state in the body. Several symptoms reveal when the body is overly acidic, such as waking in the morning with a sour taste in the mouth, anxiety, loss of tooth enamel, and fingernails that chip or break. You can also self-test your acidity levels using pH test strips available at health stores.

There are several causes of over-acidity, but the most common is the Standard American Diet (SAD), which is high in acid-forming foods such as meat, bread, pasta, and sugar. Aspartame and monosodium glutamate—also part of the SAD— also promote chronic acidity. Foods that promote an alkaline state include vegetables, some fruits, some legumes, salt, and caffeine. (Caffeine has other properties of concern to health, which I discuss later in this chapter under "Stimulants"). Conditions associated with over-acidity include constipation, liver or kidney weakness, mineral deficiencies, overeating, use of some medications, and negative emotions.[2]

Once a body is in an acidic state, the recommended dietary protocol is to eat a higher ratio of alkaline foods for a time. Dr. William Howard Hay, an early 20th-century pioneer in acid/alkaline diets, recommended one that is 20 percent acid-forming to 80 percent alkaline-forming. Today, opinions vary. I recommend a 70 percent alkaline diet to re-balance the body, in particular after an illness or for anyone who has cancer. The Alkaline Diet is in Appendix 3.

Several factors influence how alkaline our diet should be ongoing. Annemarie Colbin states: "The correct proportion will vary with each metabolism, the amount of physical activity, other foods eaten earlier and also the depth of deep breathing which alkalizes the body."[3] Physical activity plays a complex role in acid-alkaline balance. Michelle Schoffro Cook, nutritionist and doctor of natural medicine, explains: "Exercise, done properly, also helps to counter acidity in the body. It gives acid wastes another way out of the body—through sweat [however] it's important to avoid over exercising, which can increase lactic acid formation and contribute to an acidic state in the body."[4] This raises an important issue for those who do not sweat easily: there could be a greater risk of acidity from exercise. As noted previously, it is alkalizing to deep breathe, which explains why this is a health-promoting practice, whether or not one is exercising.

An over-alkaline state is rare but can occur after hyperventilating or extended vomiting. Eating only fruits and vegetables can cause a temporary alkaline excess. In this state, according to Annemarie Colbin, our bodies will prompt us to eat acidic foods, such as sweets or starches, e.g., cookies, bread, chips.[5] However, this does not mean that every time we crave these foods, we are over-alkaline. There are other reasons for such cravings that require assessment and specific therapeutic protocols, as outlined in Chapter 14.

Anti-Inflammatory

Most illness and disease involve excess inflammation. Before illness strikes, there are several warning signs of inflammation in the body, including abdominal bloating, water retention, sinus congestion, frequent colds, mucous in stools, high blood pressure, joint swelling, and high cholesterol. Often, the underlying issue is intestinal inflammation, which impairs the critical functions of digestion, absorption, and elimination, and in turn, other body functions. It is in this way that inflammation manifests anywhere in the body but has its roots in intestinal health. Inflammation triggers include the wrong diet for individual needs, viral or bacterial infections, imbalanced gut flora, parasites, and toxic accumulation from chemicals or heavy metals.

Diet can reduce inflammation anywhere in the body by first addressing it in the digestive tract. The Anti-Inflammatory Diet (Appendix 4) eases stress on digestion to allow the healing process to begin. It may be needed temporarily or on a long-term basis. I repeatedly see dramatic results with clients who follow the Anti-Inflammatory Diet:

M.G., a 60-year-old female client, had abdominal bloating, chronic diarrhea, occasional mucous in her stool, and very low energy. She was concerned about some weight loss, but medical tests had found nothing of concern. When she followed the Anti-Inflammatory Diet, her symptoms were soon reduced, her energy increased, and she gained some weight. She continued on this diet while completing healing protocols, including avoiding foods to which she was intolerant. Due to long-term damage to her digestive tract, this way of eating was advisable for her in the long term. At age 65, she returned to enjoying an active life, including frequent travel.

The Anti-Inflammatory Diet supports healing in the digestive tract during the transition from the Standard American Diet (SAD) to a good quality diet (see Chapter 7).

Immune Boosting

Those who have a disease, such as cancer, or who are recovering from gastric surgery, will have weakened immune systems. Symptoms that signal weakened or stressed immunity include frequent colds, infections, swollen glands, or swelling under the armpits. To boost immunity, use the Anti-inflammatory Diet and daily consumption of "juiced" vegetables and fruits. Juicing involves a special machine to extract only the juice from raw fruits and vegetables that preserves nutrients and plant enzymes, while eliminating roughage that might cause gastric upset. Juiced fruits and vegetables retain all their vital energy and nutrition, but are easier to digest than the raw, whole form.

Juicing provides the most benefit if the source is quality fruits and vegetables—ideally fresh and organic. Frequency is also important; for those with severe health issues, twice daily may be required. My recommended juicing formulas for immune support are:

Apple, orange, carrot, ginger, whole lemon (with peel)

Bok choy, collard greens, beet greens, kale, tomato, cucumber, carrots, onion

Low Glycemic

In the 1990s, research discovered a metabolic characteristic of carbohydrates called *glycemic value*—the rate at which the body burns different starches and sugars. In the book *The Glucose Revolution: The Authoritative Guide to the Glycemic Index—The Groundbreaking Medical Discovery* by Jennie Brand-Miller PhD, we learn that there are fast- and slow-burning carbohydrates. Diets high in slow-burning carbohydrates stabilize blood sugar, while fast-burning carbs are destabilizing.[6] This system categorizes foods as having a low- or high-glycemic effect. Low-glycemic foods are slow burning, while high-glycemic foods are fast burning. Those who have trouble regulating their blood sugar—diabetics and hypoglycemics—should favour low-glycemic foods. Appendix 5: Glycemic Values of Carbohydrates provides a handy list of high- and low-glycemic foods. There are also eating patterns that promote a low-glycemic effect from foods, such as:

- Eat every two to three hours—three meals and two snacks daily.
- Avoid simple carbohydrates, such as white sugar, and starchy foods, such as potatoes.
- Limit fruits (a simple sugar) to two daily.
- Each meal and snack should include a protein, a complex carbohydrate, and a fat.
- Favour foods with a low-glycemic effect (Appendix 5).
- Ensure there are no food sensitivities. Sensitive foods can cause blood sugar imbalances. *See Chapter 8.*

These dietary steps are essential for diabetics, even those who take insulin, as this client's experience illustrates:

A.R., a type 2 diabetic, experienced dramatic results from diet change. When she consulted me, she was taking insulin injections, but still had trouble controlling her blood sugar. Her blood pressure was also high. After she followed a low-glycemic diet and eliminated foods to which she was sensitive, she cut her insulin in half. Her blood pressure also returned to normal. Her doctor was amazed and asked her what she had done. To me, this outcome was perfectly understandable. Changes in diet can have a powerful effect on serious health issues.

A low glycemic diet also addresses the condition called hypoglycemia characterized by excess fluctuations in blood sugar, often after consumption of simple carbohydrates (e.g., white sugar, fruits) and foods high in starches (e.g., potatoes, white bread). These foods trigger a rapid rise in blood sugar, accompanied by an energized feeling. However, because of inability to regulate blood sugar, it drops quickly and results in fatigue and even depression. The body signals cravings for more sugars and starches to restore the energized feeling that these foods produce, and the blood sugar roller coaster begins again. Other symptoms of hypoglycemia include being hungry soon after eating and irritable if a meal is missed. As explained in Chapter 14, this condition can be a symptom of digestive imbalances associated with a parasitic infection. I have also found that my clients with food sensitivities have heightened responses to their sensitive food(s) that manifest as hypoglycemic symptoms.

Fasting

The temporary abstention from, or reduction of, food, called fasting, has several benefits, both physical and psychological. During fasting, the digestive energies normally used to break down and absorb food are freed up to address other critical functions, such as the elimination of toxins or easing stress from multiple food intolerances. For those with severe allergic reactions, a fast can calm the body's overactive responses and reduce the severity of allergies. Fasting is highly beneficial for those with poor nutritional habits, such as overeating, skipping meals, eating while stressed, and eating poor-quality foods. As already discussed, the Standard American Diet puts enormous stress on the digestive system. Annemarie Colbin reminds us "Not eating is probably the oldest and most universal food-related healing technique. Animals routinely stop eating if they don't feel well…and human beings have also fasted when illness struck."[7] As a spiritual practice, fasting elevates mental acuity, which is associated with spiritual enlightenment. Jesus fasted in the wilderness for 40 days to bring him closer to God. Buddhist monks fast regularly for similar reasons.

There are several kinds of fasts, but two are most commonly used: water fasting and juice fasting. The water fast involves total abstention from food and, as the name suggests, allows only water. I do not recommend this approach unless the body is already functioning well. Water fasting can release toxins too quickly for the body to handle in the presence of issues such as persistent fatigue, indigestion, irregular bowel movements, and blood sugar imbalances. Since most of my clients come to me with such issues, I have never recommended this fast.

Juice fasting is easier to tolerate because there are some nutrients in the juice. It is important to include a variety of juices using both vegetables and fruits. Having only fruit juice would mean too much sugar (fruit sugar in excess has the same ill effects as white sugar) and would negate the benefits of the fast. The ideal juice fast involves freshly prepared juice from a variety of organic fruits and vegetables.

I do not recommend self-administered fasts for longer than seven days, but they can be repeated seasonally. At other times, the Digestive Balancing Diet (see Appendix 2) can be followed to continue restoring healthy function.

Raw Food

There is an entire movement around the benefits of raw food. The advocates for a raw food diet claim we should eat most of our food raw in order to receive the maximum nutrients. While it is true cooking destroys vitamins, minerals, and important enzymes in vegetables and grains, few people would agree to eating raw meat, eggs, and poultry. The risk of bacteria and parasites in animal proteins means that cooking is needed to avoid serious, even life-threatening, infections. There is a place for raw food, however. Raw vegetables contain plant enzymes that support our own enzymatic reactions. Most people should eat some raw vegetables every day. Eating salads is the easiest way to achieve this.

In some situations, raw food is not recommended. With a weakened gall bladder, irritable bowel syndrome, colitis, or Crohn's disease, raw vegetables and grains are quite irritating to the digestive tract. When these conditions are present, most vegetables eaten by the individual should be steamed to soften the fibre. Soft vegetables, such as lettuce and spinach, may be tolerated.

For those with hypothyroid function, some vegetables are better cooked than raw. Cruciferous vegetables (broccoli, cauliflower, Brussels sprouts) contain substances called goitrogens that can depress the function of the thyroid. Cooking breaks down goitrogens and eliminates their ill effects on the thyroid.

In the presence of weak digestion, eating raw nuts can produce gastrointestinal problems. Soaking the nuts in water overnight will deactivate the enzyme inhibitors that cause such problems.

Raw milk has recently become attractive to a health-conscious population because of its beneficial enzymes, which are destroyed during pasteurization. However, raw milk can contain dangerous bacteria linked to serious illness or death. Cheese made from raw milk may be okay, but it depends on the vigilance of the producer to create a safe product. Pregnant women, older adults and those with compromised immune systems are advised to avoid raw milk cheese. In Canada, it is illegal to sell raw milk, but cheese made from raw milk is available, typically at health stores.

For most of us, a mix of raw and steamed vegetables and fruits will support health. Before embracing a strict raw food diet, a consultation with a holistic nutritionist is highly recommended.

Sprouting

The sprouting of legumes, grains, nuts, and seeds has a long tradition, dating back to a time before there was full understanding that sprouts are a nutritional powerhouse. Sprouting releases the full nutritional potential of a food, while reducing less helpful properties. In *Nourishing Traditions,* Fallon and Enig explain the benefits of sprouting: "Grains, nuts, legumes and seeds are rich in enzymes but also contain enzyme inhibitors that can put great strain on the digestive system. Sprouting…deactivates enzyme inhibitors, thus making the nutrients in grains, nuts and seeds more readily available."[8]

There are healing benefits to sprouting that are unparalleled when compared to other food preparations. Alfalfa sprouts contain *saponins*—organic compounds that lower bad LDL cholesterol and stimulate the immune system. The nutrients, enzymes, and plant compounds in sprouts all support the cardiovascular system, making them highly beneficial to those with high blood pressure or heart disease. Green leafy sprouts (e.g., alfalfa, watercress) contain high levels of antioxidants that enhance protection against the effects of aging. Almost any legume and seed can be sprouted to increase the nutritional benefits related to the food.

I recommend growing your own sprouts rather than purchasing packaged sprouts at the grocery store. There have been some instances of bacterial contamination of commercial sprouts. Sprouting at home is easy and highly economical. Health stores have sprouting kits with instructions for making your own sprouts.

Fermentation

Before refrigeration was available, fermentation was used to preserve foods. Fermenting fruits and berries led to the discovery of alcoholic beverages. But there are other foods that can be fermented—not to produce alcoholic drinks—that have health benefits such as cheese, yogurt, kefir, beets, pickles (made with cucumber), sauerkraut (made with cabbage), and sourdough breads. In the Far East, fermented grains and vegetables are consumed extensively. Asians ferment soybeans to produce soy sauce, tempeh, miso, and natto. In fact, Asians consider unfermented soy an inferior food barely fit for consumption.

Fermentation enhances a food's benefits in several ways: it improves taste, keeps the food fresh without refrigeration, increases nutritional value, softens fibre, deactivates enzyme inhibitors, and partially digests the food. Fermented foods are rich in B12, a vitamin in which many people are deficient. Beneficial bacteria, lactobacilli, are produced during the fermentation of certain foods, such as milk (e.g., yogurt) and vegetables (e.g., pickled beets). It is the bacteria in fermented food that promotes balanced intestinal bacteria, which is needed for digestion of nutrients and efficient elimination of waste. Since immunity is associated with a healthy intestinal balance, resistance to illness is enhanced.

For most people, fermented foods eaten in small quantities will provide the intended benefits. Too much fermented food, however, can cause problems. In the presence of yeast infections (e.g., athlete's foot, fungus under toenails, vaginal infections), I observe that fermented foods can aggravate the condition. I advise my clients with these tendencies to avoid fermented foods temporarily.

Stimulants: A Healing Controversy

Stimulants include several foods and food constituents, such as white flour, white sugar, animal foods, alcohol, and caffeine. Here I address caffeine because there is disagreement on its benefits and risks, and because individual responses to it vary. Caffeine is found in coffee, tea, and cocoa (consumed mostly via chocolate). When taken in moderation, caffeine has benefits such as increasing alertness and enhancing metabolic rate. Annemarie Colbin notes that because caffeine is an alkaloid, it can serve a purpose to alkalize the body from a diet too high in acid-forming foods.[9] From this point of view, a cup of coffee in the morning can be viewed as an antidote for the Standard American Diet, which is rife with foods that are acid forming, such as sugar, flour, and meat. However, because of its additive properties, caffeine is often used to excess, which is when problems can arise.

Caffeine, when consumed in excess:

- Is extremely dehydrating;
- Raises blood pressure;
- Raises blood glucose levels (a risk for diabetics);
- Increases cravings for sugar;
- Triggers formation of kidney stones;
- Interferes with healing in the digestive tract;
- Induces quick energy that can later lead to fatigue (perceived energy comes from the body's struggle to adapt to increased blood levels of stress hormones).

Giving up caffeine suddenly can produce withdrawal symptoms such as headaches, disorientation, moodiness, and fatigue. Gradual reduction of caffeine-containing foods will prevent these unpleasant symptoms.

The assessment of what constitutes excess caffeine is an individual one. Some people do not tolerate any amount; others can experience negative effects with regular use of over 100 mg of caffeine per day. Typically, this relates to the liver's inability to clear caffeine from the body efficiently. If you have symptoms of liver stress (Chapter 11), coffee and other caffeine sources should be limited. A typical cup of coffee contains 120-150 mg of caffeine; however, the Center for Science in the Public Interest reports that some popular coffee outlets can deliver over 400 mg of caffeine in one large cup of coffee.[10] Depending on the variety, tea ranges from 15 to 70 mg of caffeine per cup. In comparison, chocolate has less caffeine (100 mg per 100 grams) and contains beneficial antioxidants. Chocolate is health promoting, but only when it is high in cocoa, low in sugar and has no hydrogenated oils. The problem is that most chocolate we consume is full of these ingredients. There are benefits to eating small amounts of dark chocolate lightly sweetened with fruit.

Green tea contains less caffeine than coffee and black tea and has many beneficial properties. Its antioxidant activity may repair oxidative damage to cells caused by free radicals—unstable molecules that can harm healthy cells. If free radical damage is not addressed, many diseases and conditions can result. Excess production of free radicals in the body results from toxic exposure, after prolonged strenuous exercise, and when ascending and descending during air travel. In *Prescription for Nutritional Healing*, James and Phyllis Balch reveal these benefits: "Green tea protects against cancer, lowers cholesterol levels and reduces the clotting tendency of the blood. It also shows promise as a weight loss aid because it promotes the burning of fat and helps to regulate blood sugar and insulin levels."[11]

Soothers

Various foods and herbs can soothe issues such as irritation in the digestive system, inflammation (anywhere in the body), and anxiety from psychological stress. Here are some soothing foods and their specific benefits:

Basil, spearmint, peppermint, all part of the mint family, are beneficial as digestive aids, a mild sedative, and in the treatment of headaches.

Celery juice contains a sedative that calms the nerves and helps reduce blood pressure.

Cinnamon has confirmed effects as a sedative to relieve muscle spasms and insomnia. It is also a digestive aid and improves circulation.

Chamomile and tarragon address insomnia, nervousness, and hyperactivity. When taken as tea, there is an added advantage in rotation with **sage tea**, another stress reliever that can address excess perspiration.

Dill can address flatulence and digestive disturbance.

Ginger eases stomachaches, indigestion, and nausea.

Nutmeg can be helpful in combatting diarrhea and improving intestinal tone.

Oatmeal supports the nervous system and adrenal glands, reduces cholesterol; it is a short-term tonic to address low blood pressure and is helpful during recovery from illness.

Saffron relieves inflammation.

Turkey contains tryptophan, which calms and soothes. If you want a good night's sleep, eat turkey for dinner.

Important note: Soothing foods provide the most benefit when consumed while adhering to one of the six healing diets outlined in this chapter.

Some of the information in this chapter is not new, but has unfortunately passed out of common knowledge. I believe that in North America, ancient wisdom about food and healing has been pushed aside by modern medical approaches. It is time we re-embraced the healing power of food. I believe this will prove to be our greatest hope for restoring health and being well.

Chapter Notes

1. Donna Gates, *Body Ecology Diet: Recovering Your Health and Rebuilding Your Immunity* (Carlsbad, California: Hay House Inc., 2010).

2. Ibid.

3. Annemarie Colbin, *Food and Healing*, Tenth anniversary edition (New York, New York: Ballantyne Books, 1996), 78.

4. Michelle Schoffro Cook, DMN, DAc, CNC, *The Ultimate pH Solution: Balance Your Body Chemistry to Prevent Disease and Lose Weight* (Toronto, Ontario: Harper Collins, 2008), 120.

5. Annemarie Colbin, *Food and Healing.*

6. Jennie Brand-Miller et al., *The Glucose Revolution: The Authoritative Guide to the Glycemic Index—the Groundbreaking Medical Discovery* (New York, New York: Marlowe and Company, 1996).

7. Annemarie Colbin, *Food and Healing,* 257.

8. Sally Fallon with Mary G. Enig, PhD, *Nourishing Traditions,* Revised 2nd edition (Washington, DC: New Trends Publishing Inc., 2001), 47.

9. Annemarie Colbin, *Food and Healing,* 76.

10. "Caffeine Content of Food and Drugs," *Center for Science in the Public Interest, Cspinet.org* (December 2012), accessed September 14, 2014, http://www.cspinet.org/new/cafchart.htm.

11. James Balch and Phyllis Balch, *Prescription for Nutritional Healing,* Second edition (Garden City Park, New York: Avery Publishing, 1997), 44.

13: KNOW WHEN DIET IS NOT ENOUGH

Joe has a busy life. Work, family, and social connections keep him hopping. He is always eating on the run and his meals are often takeout or fast food. He eats at his desk or in the car on his way to the next appointment. He believes that taking a multivitamin/mineral supplement will make up for his busy lifestyle and poor diet.

Joe's story is all too common in our fast-paced society. Through the discussion in this chapter, I address these critical questions: *Is Joe's use of supplements health supportive? What role do supplements play in natural healing?*

The first inkling that specific nutrients in foods were critical to health was discovered by a doctor treating scurvy-afflicted British sailors in the 1700s. By accident, this doctor discovered the sailors who ate fruits were more likely to recover from scurvy. The British navy began supplying their crews with limes, and scurvy was no longer a problem. (This is how British sailors came to be known as "limeys.") However, no one knew how limes prevented scurvy. It was not until early in the 20th century that scientists isolated specific nutrients in food (vitamins) and identified their beneficial properties. One of the first discoveries was that the muscle-wasting disease Beriberi was because of a deficiency of B1 (thiamine)—the result of eating white (polished) rice. Since then, many micronutrients have been identified, as well as their specific benefits to health. Today, supplements of micronutrients are widely used to optimize health, not only to address deficiencies.

One of the guiding principles of holistic nutrition from the Canadian School of Natural Nutrition is the "recognition that supplementation is not a substitute for wholesome, nutritious food but can be helpful in recommended form, dose and frequency."[1] Nutritional supplements of any kind—vitamins, minerals, enzymes, herbs, amino acids, glandular extracts, and homeopathic remedies—are not insurance against an unhealthy diet and lifestyle. Taking supplements without following a healthy diet is like throwing lilacs on a pile of cow manure. The manure might smell and look better, but its properties will stay the same. In the same way, supplements can make us feel better without addressing the underlying reasons for health concerns. This chapter discusses the benefits of natural supplements, and under what circumstances they support natural healing.

Diet *May* Be Enough

At one time, people believed diet alone was sufficient—that they did not need nutritional supplements to maintain health. The North American medical community held this position until 2001, when a review article in the *Journal of the American Medical Association* (JAMA) stated that supplements were likely needed because hardly anyone was eating "properly."[2] More recently, medical oncologist Dr. David Agus, in his book *The End of Illness,* claims the opposite—that nutritional supplements are not needed. He maintains that all we have to do is eat real food and avoid processed foods.[3] I take issue with this position for a couple of reasons: it is difficult to know if "real" food, such as fruits and vegetables, contains the nutrients we expect. Tragically, nutrient-deficient food is readily available and cheaper than quality food. During illness and chronic health conditions, nutritional supplements are often essential to recovery.

In my clinical experience, diet *may* be enough for *some* people. In Part I of this book, I discuss the challenges to maintaining a healthy diet. Our food can be nutrient deficient and contain health-damaging sugar, fats, chemicals, and additives. Environmental toxins in the air and water further burden our bodies' ability to function optimally. In North America, where most of the population has enough food to eat, these challenges make nutritional deficiencies more common than we would expect. I see this repeatedly with my clients. Deficiencies in vitamins and minerals can occur at a subclinical level, meaning medical blood testing does not consider the deficiencies sufficient to cause illness. However, a minor deficiency in one or more nutrients can make it difficult to be well and to prevent serious illness.

The Case for Nutritional Supplements

Research into the value of nutritional supplements has a relatively short history. The pioneer of vitamin supplementation was Nobel laureate Linus Pauling, who in the 1960s concluded that vitamin C was a cure for the common cold. Although this suggestion proved to be overly optimistic, vitamin C supplementation is now widely viewed as important. Humans do not manufacture this vitamin, so it must come through diet or supplements. Vitamin D supplementation is also considered essential, in particular for those living in northern climates.

Knowledge about supplementing with vitamins such as C and D comes from research only in the past 50 years. There are various methods to study the benefits of vitamins and minerals: laboratory, animal experimentation, epidemiology (the study of populations), clinical trials, and clinical experience. No one method has proven ideal in the study of micronutrients.

In the laboratory, the action of vitamins can be assessed in a test tube. The antioxidant effects of micronutrients such as vitamins C and E and beta-carotene are well established by this kind of research. However, this is theoretical knowledge that does not prove how they work in the human body.

Supplement research with lab animals has found potential benefits for humans. Compared to other research methods, the results may be more reliable because the animals' food and environment are controlled and outside factors eliminated. However, there is doubt whether the results with animals can be generalized to humans. In addition, most of the animal research has focused on the role of supplements in preventing or treating illness and disease, rather than supporting health and wellness. Researchers cannot ask a lab rat how well it feels.

Epidemiological, or population, studies have produced variable and often conflicting results. Some studies found benefit, while others did not. To illustrate the challenges in making meaningful connections between supplements and health, there are the diverse findings about vitamin E supplements. The Nurses' Health Study, an eight-year follow-up of 87,000 middle-aged women, concluded that vitamin E supplements, but not dietary vitamin E, were associated with lower risk of cardiovascular disease.[4] In contrast, a well-publicized Finnish study in the 1990s determined that supplementary vitamin E was related to an increased risk for prostate cancer and lung cancer.[5] A review of numerous studies by researchers at Oregon State University in 2007 discussed the various benefits of vitamin E: "In lab, animal or human studies, there is evidence that vitamin E can reduce oxidative stress, inhibit formation of atherosclerotic lesions, slow aortic thickening, lower inflammation, and reduce platelet adhesion."[6] These widely varying conclusions about one vitamin supplement leave many puzzled what to believe.

Practitioners have a wealth of clinical experience showing the benefit of nutritional supplements, but this is seldom seen as reliable scientific evidence. In truth, practitioners with clients who benefit from supplements cannot be 100 percent certain that supplements made the critical difference. Ironically, it is from observations in clinical practice that modern medicine built its current knowledge about diagnosis and treatment. This question remains: at what point is evidence from clinical practice sufficient proof of the benefit of supplements? I suspect it will be when the weight of evidence becomes so overwhelming that it can no longer be discounted.

Flawed Research on Nutritional Supplements

The challenges in making conclusions from research on foods and diet are discussed in Chapter 3. Research on specific nutrients has similar challenges. I have identified six flaws in research on nutrients that make the findings of such studies potentially unreliable:

- Nutrients do not work in isolation, but in synergistic ways with other nutrients.
- It is difficult to control for other factors affecting health.
- Causal links are made between a nutrient and a health issue when their presence is merely associated.
- Ethical issues arise when studies deny humans needed nutrients.
- Synthetic or partial formulas are used that do not provide intended benefit.
- Dosages are used that do not provide therapeutic benefit.

These research flaws each have their own impact on research findings, as the following discussion illustrates.

Nutrients are synergistic: We would never expect to thrive if we ate only one food, even if it were hailed as a miracle food. The same is true of micronutrients; they provide benefits in combination with other vitamins and minerals. For example, to be effective, vitamin E needs adequate levels of vitamin C and the mineral selenium. The body produces a powerful antioxidant called glutathione from specific nutrients—vitamins C, E, alpha-lipoic acid, and an amino acid called cysteine. Calcium promotes bone development, but only in combination with other minerals (magnesium, manganese, boron, phosphorus, vanadium) and Vitamin D. Studies claiming that one nutrient will make a difference to human health run counter to what is known about nutrition and human health.

Not controlling other factors affecting health: To isolate the effects of specific nutrients, researchers must allow for other influences such as diet, environment, emotions, and underlying health issues. As discussed in Chapter 3, this is extremely difficult to accomplish in human studies, which typically involve self-reports from participants about their health behaviours—hardly as reliable as direct observation.

Making causal links between a nutrient and a health issue: Studies want to prove that a nutrient *causes* a specific health outcome, and perhaps it is not surprising when they find such links. A prime example of this is a population study that ended in 2011, which concluded that taking a multivitamin supplement was related to a higher rate of death. This study tracked 39,000 women aged 55 to 69 for 19 years and found higher death rates among supplement users. The news headline read: "Study links vitamins to higher death rates in women."[7] The implication in the headline is that taking supplements *causes* higher death rates, or at least that the vitamins provide no benefit. However, there are other explanations for the study's findings. Perhaps the women who took the supplements were already in poor health. People with an illness are more apt to seek extra nutritional support than healthy individuals. Also, during the 19 years, many of the women would have reached their life expectancies—supplements cannot save people from dying. Unfortunately, numerous studies observe an association between events or conditions and mistakenly conclude there is a direct cause and effect between those events or conditions. This confuses people about the role of nutritional supplements and is a disservice to nutritional science.

Ethics of denying nutrients: The randomized double-blind study is the most respected research method, and the one used to study pharmaceutical drugs. This method randomly divides participants into two groups. One takes the nutrient under study, while the other, the control group, does not. Neither the participants nor the researchers know who is in which group—hence the term "double-blind." As noted in Chapter 2, the ethics of this method in nutrition research with humans have been questioned because denying nutrients could pose a health risk. Dr. Abram Hoffer and Linus Pauling proposed human studies use a natural control group made up of those who voluntarily withdraw from the study.[8] This provides a group for comparison purposes, while allowing for the individual right of choice. I am not aware of studies using natural control groups.

Formulas that are not health promoting: Synthetic forms of nutrients are often used in studies, even though they do not provide the same benefit as natural forms. A prime example is the use of synthetic vitamin E or *dl-alpha tocopherol* instead of the natural form, *d-alpha tocopherol*. Also, to accurately study vitamin E, the formula should include mixed *tocopherols* and *tocotrienols*. Few studies do this. Vitamin C as ascorbic acid is not a natural form, either. To do its important work, vitamin C must have its co-factors, called bioflavonoids—rutin, quercetin, and hesperidin. A study involving only ascorbic acid is not evaluating a truly beneficial supplement. The source and quality of supplements is also an issue. Tablets have binders and excipients to hold the pill together and to extend the supplement's shelf life. These can be harmful to health in some individuals. It is also possible that such tablets are not fully absorbed.

Dosage not at a therapeutic level: Studies often use the Recommended Daily Allowance (RDA) for a supplement that does not provide therapeutic benefit. Consider again the 2011 study assessing the impact of multivitamin supplements on women's health.[9] By focusing on death rates, the study attributed therapeutic value to supplements with RDA-level nutrients that are intended as supportive to health. Few people realize that the RDA of vitamin C, at 60 mg, is the daily intake required to prevent scurvy. To be therapeutic, vitamin C must be taken at doses of several thousand milligrams. The therapeutic level of vitamin E is anywhere from 800 to 3200 IU, four to eight times higher than the dosage used in most vitamin E trials. The previously mentioned 2007 review of vitamin E studies made this conclusion: "Generations of studies may be largely meaningless because new research has demonstrated that the levels of this micronutrient necessary to reduce oxidative stress are far higher than those that have been commonly used in clinical trials."[10]

To illustrate how flawed research can appear valid, there was the large scale, well-publicized Finnish clinical trial ending in 1994 that concluded vitamin E and beta-carotene supplementation increased the risk of cancer. The study group comprised male smokers who continued to indulge in their unhealthy habit. When vitamin E failed to help these health-challenged participants, researchers concluded that the vitamin E caused further health problems.[11] Complementary physician Michael Schachter points to several problems making any conclusions from this study. The dosage of vitamin E and beta-carotene was much lower than is required for cancer prevention. In addition, in the scientific community, Finland is widely considered a poor site for cancer/nutrition studies because of the Finns' high rate of smoking and alcohol consumption and low levels of dietary selenium because of nutrient-deficient crops. Vitamin E is only effective in cancer prevention in combination with adequate amounts of selenium.[12] Despite the shortcomings in the Finnish study, other researchers and the media routinely cite it as proof that supplements are not helpful, and perhaps even harmful. When research makes big headlines (such as the Finnish study), it is important to assess the study's methods with a critical eye before accepting its findings.

Being Well with Nutritional Supplements

Nutritional supplements have a place in restoring healthy balance, as *adjuncts* to a healthy diet, lifestyle, and a toxin-free environment. If diet and lifestyle are addressed and health concerns persist, only then should supplements be considered. As discussed in Chapter 10, natural healing is advanced by taking supplements either therapeutically or supportively. Therapeutic use of supplements relies on careful attention to dosage, frequency and synergy of various nutrients, and ideally is supervised by a holistic practitioner trained in orthomolecular nutrition, which is about correcting imbalances or deficiencies based on individual biochemistry. Supportive supplements are adjuncts to therapeutic protocols, although there is sometimes a fine line between supportive and therapeutic use. Before discussing situations when supplements aid healing in either of these ways, it is important to recognize the third way to use of supplements—palliatively.

The story of Joe in the introduction to this chapter is an example of palliative supplementation. He used supplements to make up for a poor diet and stress from overwork. Palliative use of supplements may ease symptoms but fail to address the underlying cause, prolonging or preventing the healing process. For this reason, I discourage palliative use, with a few exceptions. With a diagnosed chronic condition that natural healing can only partially address, a palliative supplement will improve the quality of life. For example, certain supplements can ease the pain from degeneration in the joints. I will not comment further on palliative uses here because my focus is on healing.

When to Use Supplements

From my clinical experience and study of reliable research, I identify several situations in which supplements are beneficial, either therapeutically or supportively. As already mentioned, the line between a therapeutic and supportive use can be a fuzzy one. The following situations may warrant supplementation.

Vegetarian Diet
Vegetarian proteins (legumes, nuts, seeds) are typically deficient in B12 and often iron. Strict vegans, who consume no animal proteins, should consider supplementation with these micronutrients.

Winters in northern climates

The lack of sun exposure during winter in northern latitudes increases the need for supplementary vitamin D. The skin, when exposed to sunlight, produces this vitamin, which is more like a hormone. In addition, food does not contain the same nutrient levels during winter due to long transit times. Northern dwellers must supplement with vitamin D in winter. The high incidence of cancer in northern latitudes may be related to low vitamin D levels in the body during winter. For some individuals, especially older adults, broad nutritional support (e.g., multi-vitamin/mineral) is typically needed during winter.

During weight loss

A reduction in calories to achieve weight loss also means a reduction in nutrients. Over time, this can lead to nutrient deficiencies. Among dieters, even minor nutrient deficits can trigger cravings that seriously derail their weight-loss efforts. For those attempting to lose weight, I recommend, at minimum, a multivitamin/mineral complex. Other nutrients may be needed, but this is ideally determined through a holistic assessment of the individual's current and past diet, dieting history, metabolic function, and overall health status.

With Aging

As discussed in Chapter 10, the journey to being unwell is hastened by free radical damage in the body. Tufts University in Boston has conducted extensive research on the relationship between aging and free radicals. Tuft's e-book *Antioxidants* states:

> The damage [from free radicals], called oxidative stress, can accumulate and contribute to the development of several chronic diseases, including cardiovascular disease, diabetes, and cancer, as well as age-related conditions, such as macular degeneration, cataracts, and neurodegenerative diseases such as Alzheimer's. Antioxidants are compounds that prevent free radicals from damaging the cells of your body.[13]

In Table 1, note that two antioxidants decline with age: alpha-lipoic acid and coenzyme Q10. The former is critical in the body's production of the antioxidant glutathione and the latter is essential to a healthy cardiovascular system. Research on vitamin C determined our bodies do not produce this vitamin. Therefore, to maintain health, we must take it in from diet or supplements. In 1992, a population survey in the United States found that those who took vitamin C supplements also had less risk of dying of cardiovascular disease.[14] Tufts also quotes several studies showing that antioxidants help reduce the risk of stroke.[15]

With aging, the ability to absorb nutrients is often compromised because of a decline in bodily functions, either digestion or metabolism or both. Minerals are the nutrients most often affected by malabsorption. Supplementation with a multi-mineral complex is beneficial; this is contrary to the popular notion that only calcium supplementation is important.

Dysfunction in digestion or metabolism

When digestion is not working efficiently, digestive enzymes and probiotic supplements are beneficial and often required to restore good health. Long-term illness and age can reduce digestive ability to where such supplements are needed ongoing. There are also specific vitamins and minerals that support digestive processes. For example, B6, inositol, and choline all support the liver. Blood sugar imbalances can be stabilized by supplementing with chromium and niacin. With metabolic dysfunction, it is advisable to use supplements under the advice and supervision of a holistic health practitioner.

During Illness

In the presence of viruses, bacterial infections, and chronic illnesses the immune system often requires support. This is when naturally occurring free radicals can be helpful. The body produces free radicals as a part of the immune response to attack by viruses and bacteria. Naturopath John Matsen explains how free radicals can also serve a useful purpose in activating hormones and enzymes, but when these same free radicals are produced in excess, we need antioxidants to neutralize them.[16] A broad range of vitamins and minerals support recovery from illness. They fall under two categories—immune builders and immune boosters.

Immune builders include the antioxidant vitamins C, E, and D, some B vitamins, the minerals selenium and iodine, specific amino acids, and enzymes. The most critical of these and the agents that deplete them from the body are presented in Table 1: Key Antioxidants: Sources and Enemies. Given the extent to which we are exposed to these "enemies" through diet and the environment, it is very easy to be depleted of immune builders. During recovery from illness, supplementing them is essential to healing.

Immune boosters include herbs such as echinacea, astragalus, goldenseal, ginger, curcumin, and ginseng. Several varieties of mushroom (reishi, shitake, and maitake) are also significant immune boosters. Caution must be taken in using boosters because they can interact in unwanted ways with prescription medications. Those with autoimmune disease (e.g., rheumatoid arthritis, Crohn's) are also not advised to use immune boosters because they can stimulate the already overly active immune response and further aggravate the disease.

Toxic Accumulation

An overload of toxins puts a great strain on the body, and this could be anywhere, depending on where the toxins have accumulated. With absorption of toxins, the liver becomes overburdened and, instead of clearing them from the body, deposits them somewhere in the body, such as the lining of intestines, fat cells, nerve endings, or joints. Toxic overload from chemicals and heavy metals depletes specific nutrients, in particular the very antioxidants that are needed for an immune response to the toxins. Supplementation is often the only way to replace these lost nutrients. With certain degrees of toxicity, therapeutic levels of nutritional supplements, herbs, and homeopathic remedies are essential to help the body detoxify. See Chapter 15 for more on detoxification.

TABLE 1: Key Antioxidants: Sources and Enemies

Micronutrient and Benefit	Sources	Enemies
Vitamin A (Beta carotene) Protects against UVA damage and cataracts	Orange fruits and vegetables, broccoli, green leafy vegetables	Polyunsaturated fats, Alcohol, ASA, Antacids, Cholesterol-lowering drugs
Vitamin C Anti-viral Anti-bacterial	Red sweet peppers, berries, kiwifruit, green leafy vegetables	Water, Cooking, Oxygen, ASA, Cough Syrup, Tobacco, Fluoride, Toxicity: Aluminum, Lead, Mercury
Vitamin E Increases resistance to infection. Reduces damage caused by stress	Nuts, seeds, wheat germ, fish liver oils	Heat, Oxygen, Freezing, Food processing, Iron, Chlorinated water Toxicity: Mercury
Vitamin B6 Stimulates production of antibodies	Whole grains and meats	Long storage, Canning, Cooking, Freezing, Food processing, Alcohol Toxicity: Cadmium
Zinc Eliminates toxins Anti-viral Anti-bacterial	Animal proteins, oysters, mushrooms, whole grains	Caffeine, Low stomach acid, Digestive disorders, Aging, Oral contraceptives Toxicity: Copper
Selenium Free radical fighter Reduces inflammation	Garlic, onions, tuna, herring, broccoli, egg yolks, red grapes	Food processing, Oral contraceptives Toxicity: Mercury
Alpha-Lipoic Acid "Pinch hits" for other antioxidants & maximizes their effect	Some kinds of mushrooms	Aging
Coenzyme Q10 Aids heart respiration	Small amounts in a variety of foods	Aging, Cholesterol-lowering drugs

Medications

Medications can increase the risk of deficiencies of specific vitamins and minerals. Pelton and LaValle[17] identify several medications with nutrient depletions:

- Laxatives (*bisacodyl*) deplete potassium
- Birth control pills deplete folic acid, several B vitamins, selenium and zinc
- Salicylates (aspirin) deplete vitamin B5, vitamin C, folic acid, calcium, iron, potassium, and sodium
- NSAIDs (non-steroidal anti-inflammatory drugs, e.g., ibuprofen) deplete folic acid
- Antidepressants (tricyclic) deplete CoQ10 and vitamin B2
- Thyroid medications (synthetic) deplete iron
- Proton pump inhibitors deplete vitamin B12
- Statin medications deplete coenzyme Q10
- Diuretics (blood thinners) deplete minerals, in particular potassium

Other drugs can contribute to nutrient depletion. Chemotherapy drugs impair the intestinal lining through which nutrients are absorbed; this can lead to a wide range of deficiencies. Those who take multiple medications may require supplements, but ideally, a holistic practitioner should assess for the specific needs.

It is unfortunate many people decide what supplements to take based on a book, news report, or TV program. These sources provide general information that may or may not apply to individual needs. To determine the need for supplements, it is advisable to seek the advice of a holistic health professional.

Criteria for Choosing a Supplement

There is great variation among supplements on the market and this affects their intended benefit. The adage "you get what you pay for" may apply, but I have found that price is not always the best indicator of value. I have three criteria for selecting supplements that will support the healing process: dosage, quality, and formulation.

Dosage

Determining the dosage of nutrients is essential to provide the intended benefit. The understanding of optimal dosage is an area of health practice known as orthomolecular medicine or orthomolecular health. Orthomolecular Medicine Online defines the field as one that "aims to restore the optimum environment of the body by correcting imbalances or deficiencies based on individual biochemistry, using substances natural to the body such as vitamins, minerals, amino acids, trace elements and fatty acids."[18]

An orthomolecular approach is the foundation of one of the guiding principles of holistic nutrition: "each person is biochemically distinct and has unique nutritional needs." This means that supplement dosages must be determined on an individual basis and ideally by a practitioner who is trained in orthomolecular health. Often the determination of the ideal dosage is based on research and clinical experience, but ideally the practitioner bases recommendations on individual needs.

Blood tests are the primary method for identifying nutrient deficiencies, but in Canada, medical doctors are currently the only practitioner allowed to order blood tests. As a holistic health practitioner, I use two assessment tools that point reliably to deficiencies: nutritional symptomatology (discussed in Chapter 11) and Bioenergetic Evaluation (Appendix 1). Nutritional symptomatology is the science of symptom patterns that, besides revealing functional health problems, can point to low levels of vitamins, minerals, proteins, and essential fatty acids. The Bioenergetic Evaluation is a test through the body's meridians, representing its energy pathways, in clinical use for over 50 years, with studies also backing up its effectiveness. The body's energy responds in such a way that supplements and dosages can be determined. In my clinical practice, I find this testing to be an extremely reliable method for determining a suitable supplementation plan.

I have purposely not given dosage recommendations for any supplement. There are too many variables affecting individual health to make specific recommendations in a book. Taking advice from a book represents a risk of either taking too much or too little to provide the intended benefit. A prime example is the commonly recommended dosage of 1200 to 1500 mg calcium for those at risk of osteoporosis. However, this amount is supposed to come from a combination of diet and supplements. No one would need 1200 mg of calcium from a supplement because no diet would be totally devoid of this mineral. How much calcium typically comes from diet? My analysis indicates you could receive 630 mg of calcium by consuming three green vegetables, one orange vegetable, twelve almonds, three ounces of canned salmon, a cup of rice, and one dairy food or alternative (e.g., rice or almond milk). However, food quality will affect nutrient levels, such as calcium.

There is evidence that people who supplement with calcium may take too much. A large 2008 study found a link between calcium supplementation of 1000 mg per day and increased risk of kidney stones and cardiovascular events, and with no reduction in osteoporosis and bone fractures.[19] Perhaps as a result, newer guidelines are for the Recommended Daily Allowance of 1200 mg of calcium to come from a combination of diet and supplements.[20] Supplements should fill in the gap not supplied by diet, which, according to the example in the previous paragraph would be approximately 600mg calcium per day.

I have concerns about taking calcium-only supplements because it is well known that bone building requires a combination of nutrients: calcium, magnesium, manganese, boron, and vitamin D. A calcium-only supplement could create a mineral imbalance in the body. Dosage of mineral supplements, indeed of any nutrient, should be based on average daily intake from diet and the individual's ability to absorb these nutrients. Assessments of nutrient balance are available in consultation with a holistic nutritionist. I address dosage concerns about other supplements in the next section.

Can We Overdose on Supplements?

Supplemental vitamins, minerals, and essential fatty acids will not cause harm when taken responsibly. However, it is important to be aware of the maximum dosages of certain nutrients and micronutrients, after which there is no benefit, and the potential to create imbalances. I have just discussed the potential for taking too much calcium from supplements. Some vitamin/mineral supplements on the market may have an excessive amount of minerals that can be harmful if taken over long periods. Often the excess can be inadvertent when taking several supplements with some similar ingredients. According to Health Canada, the currently accepted upper limits for daily intake of some key minerals are:[21]

Manganese	11 mg
Zinc	40 mg
Iron	45 mg
Boron	20 mg
Copper	10,000 mcg
Vanadium	1.8 mg

Fat-soluble vitamins such as A, D, and E must be taken with caution. Unlike water-soluble vitamins, these vitamins are not easily excreted by the body if too much is ingested. When taken to excess for long periods, there can be ill effects. There is some debate about the upper limit allowable for each of these vitamins. Upper limits range varies depending on the source:

Vitamin A	25,000 IU to 50,000 IU
Vitamin E	400 to 800 IU
Vitamin D	1000 to 5000 IU

Upper limits can also vary because under certain health situations, more of these vitamins might be needed on a short-term basis to make up for identified deficiencies. As mentioned in this chapter, those living in northern climates need additional vitamin D during the winter. This is when the higher dosage of 5000 IU would be beneficial.

My dosage rule of thumb is this: more is not always better. Individual needs and circumstances must be considered. When health is compromised, the optimal dosage to provide therapeutic benefit can be higher than is recommended above. In *Beyond Antibiotics: Healthier Options for Families*, Dr. Michael A. Schmidt's commentary on vitamin C illustrates the variations in what is considered the ideal dosage: "Vitamin C has a very wide margin of safety. Dr. Linus Pauling, the pioneer advocate of vitamin C, recommended between 1000 mg and 18,000 mg daily, while Dr. Roger Williams suggested 1500 mg. During times of infection, this can easily be increased to 10,000 or 20,000 mg per day."[22]

Quality

Supplements vary widely in manufacturing (purity of ingredients), source of ingredients, and form (tablets, caps, liquid, powder). These quality issues affect the supplements' bioactivity—how well they are absorbed and used by the body. Supplements can contain fillers, binders, lubricants, colours, and preservatives, which can reduce their intended benefits and even harm health.

In the book *Never Be Sick Again: Health Is a Choice, Learn How to Choose It*, Raymond Francis claims that his own chemical hypersensitivity was made worse by poor-quality supplements. Even seemingly, benign ingredients approved for supplements may not be health supportive. Supplements containing preservatives, alcohol, and sugar or other sweeteners can promote acidity in the body and increase the risk for developing health problems.[23]

Supplement additives I believe to be of most concern include the artificial colour tartrazine (aka yellow dye #5), and the preservatives BHT and BHA. My concerns about their specific health risks are outlined in Chapter 2. Large tablets that are yellow or orange are apt to contain tartrazine. Any tablet could contain the preservatives BHT or BHA. I have identified sensitivities to these additives with many of my clients.

The supplement's form can make a big difference to its benefit. Research in the late 1980s found that some supplements in tablet form were not dissolving and therefore not providing any benefit.[24] To avoid the possibility that a tablet is not dissolving, I recommend supplements in capsule or powder form. These are less likely to contain potentially harmful binders, fillers, and preservatives. I would also caution against supplements in liquid form because they usually contain a preservative. I have three standards for a supplement form of good quality: powder or capsule form, high standards of manufacturing, and forms closest to nature. Less expensive supplements are more likely to contain harmful additives. However, price is not the only criterion. Companies who advertise heavily may not spend enough on their ingredients. I also find that supplements from direct sales companies can be pricey without providing higher value. Before buying a supplement, I recommend visiting the company website to be assured of the source of ingredients and manufacturing methods. Holistic practitioners can also recommend the best quality products.

Formulas

Vitamins and minerals in supplements come in a variety of formulas that affect their bioactivity and benefit. The mineral calcium is available in various forms: carbonate, oxide, citrate, fumarate, malate, microcrystalline forms, and chelated (calcium attached to an amino acid—listed as aspartate). Carbonate and oxide forms are the least well absorbed, while the others are better to varying degrees. If you are taking a carbonate form, a higher dosage is needed to receive benefit. With microcrystalline and chelated forms, lower milligrams are needed.

To illustrate the importance of formulas, a research study on postmenopausal women found that those supplementing with potassium citrate had gains in bone mineral density, while those supplementing with potassium chloride did not. The researchers of this study conducted at the University of Basel in Switzerland concluded that the alkaline form of potassium—the citrate form—could be more effective in promoting bone mass.[25]

Vitamin C is often sold as ascorbic acid. However, vitamin C does not occur in this form in nature. As I have already stated, this vitamin is present in food in association with bioflavonoids. To ensure benefit, vitamin C supplements should always include bioflavonoids. Simple ascorbic acid may not provide the intended benefit and, with some people, can cause gastric upset. For maximum utilization and minimal gastric upset, vitamin C is available in a buffered form with minerals such as calcium, magnesium, and potassium.

The widest variety in formulas and benefit can be seen in the multiple or multivitamin/mineral supplements. In 2003, biochemist Lyle MacWilliam published a resource book evaluating 213 multivitamin/mineral supplements in North America according to several key factors: bioavailability, potency, antioxidants, cardiac support, metabolic support, bone health, and potential toxicities.[26] When MacWilliam released the first edition of his book, he had no affiliations with supplement manufacturing or sales. However, he eventually joined the medical advisory board of the company producing his top-ranked vitamin/mineral product. The book's subsequent editions could be biased to this company's product, but based on my knowledge of supplement quality I still find his work helpful in the selection of a multivitamin/mineral supplement.

Issues with Supplements

Even if the supplement is from a natural source without potential allergens, there can still be unwanted reactions. Rather than assuming the supplement is harmful, reactions may tell us something about the health status of the individual. Here are some common reactions and possible reasons:

I have allergic reactions to vitamin C.

This reaction is more likely either an allergy to one of the excipients used in the tablet's manufacture, or a sensitivity to corn. As Dr. Michael Schmidt states, some brands of vitamin C are derived from corn.[27] Many vitamin C supplements are derived from citrus and are problematic for those who are sensitive to these fruits.

That calcium supplement made me sick.

According to Dr. John Matsen, this can point to malabsorption of minerals. There may low stomach acid, a condition that results in poor mineral uptake.[28] Steps must be taken to restore efficient digestion.

That chlorophyll supplement made me nauseated.

Chlorophyll is the green pigment found in plants that, as a supplement, supports detoxification. When a chlorophyll supplement results in nausea, this could point to weakness in the liver's detoxification functions. Dr. Bernard Jensen explains how a sluggish liver can lead to poor breakdown of fats, both fat-soluble vitamins and essential fatty acids.[29] Thus, reactions to chlorophyll supplements can point to poor nutrient absorption. Symptoms of liver stress, discussed in Chapter 11, would also be present, and the supportive steps described there would be required.

I take supplements. Why don't I feel better?

Apart from the quality of supplements and the specific examples just noted, there are other reasons for poor responses. One of the most common reasons is the use of supplements as the only health-promoting activity, as illustrated in Joe's story at the beginning of this chapter. Being well comes from *all* our choices to do with diet, as well as physical and emotional environment. A poor response to supplements can also point to sensitivity to one or more of the ingredients. This is most apt to occur with herbal ingredients. Using Bioenergetic Evaluation, I have determined that if we do not tolerate even one ingredient in a supplement, we may receive no benefit and may even experience ill effects. Some herbs can depress or stimulate the action of prescription medications. Care must always be taken in using herbs while taking prescriptions. It is important to rule out illness and disease before taking supplements, which could mask symptoms of the illness and delay its diagnosis.

Despite some controversy and confusion about nutritional supplements, I know them to be a valuable tool in the healing process, when used appropriately. Therapeutic and supportive use aids healing, while palliative use only relieves symptoms. Supplements may only become therapeutic when given at specific dosages, frequency, and in quality formulas. Often therapeutic supplements are only available from a holistic health practitioner who knows how to administer them for the intended benefit.

Chapter Notes

1. "Nutrition Scope of Practice," *Canadian School of Natural Nutrition, Csnn.ca,* accessed August 20, 2014, www.csnn.ca/holistic-nutrition-industry/.

2 .Kathleen M. Fairfield, MD, and R.H. Fletcher, MD, "Vitamins for chronic disease prevention in adults: scientific review," *Journal of the American Medication Association* 287 no.23 (2002): 3127-3129, accessed August 15, 2014, doi:10.1001/jama.287.23.3127.

3. Dr. David B. Agus, *The End of Illness* (New York, New York: Free Press, 2011).

4. M.J. Stampfer et al., "A prospective study of vitamin E consumption and risk of coronary disease in women," *New England Journal of Medicine* 328 (1993): 1444-1449, accessed August 18, 2014, http://www.nejm.org/doi/pdf/10.1056/NEJM199305203282003.

5. Alpha-Tocopherol Beta Carotene Cancer Prevention Study Group, "The Effect of Vitamin E and Beta Carotene on the Incidence of Lung Cancer and Other Cancers in Male Smokers," *New England Journal of Medicine* 330 (April 1994): 1029-1035, accessed August 20, 2014, http://www.nejm.org/doi/full/10.1056/NEJM199404143301501.

6. "Vitamin E Trials Fatally Flawed," *Science Daily, Sciencedaily.com* (September 2007), accessed August 20, 2014, http://www.sciencedaily.com/releases/2007/09/070923193622.htm.

7. Angela Mulholland, "Study links vitamins to higher death rates in women," *CTVNews.ca* (October 11, 2011), accessed August 20, 2014, http://www.ctvnews.ca/study-links-vitamins-to-higher-death-rates-in-women-1.709663.

8. Dr. Abram Hoffer, MD, FRCP with Linus Pauling, PhD, *Healing Cancer: Complementary Vitamin and Drug Treatments* (Toronto, Ontario: Canadian College of Naturopathic Medicine Press, 2004).

9. Angela Mulholland, "Study links vitamins to higher death rates in women."

10. "Vitamin E Trials Fatally Flawed," *Science Daily.*

11. Alpha-Tocopherol Beta Carotene Cancer Prevention Study Group, "The Effect of Vitamin E and Beta Carotene on the Incidence of Lung Cancer and Other Cancers in Male Smokers."

12. Michael Schachter, MD, "Integrative Medicine: The Vitamin E-Beta Carotene Cancer Study in Finland," *Healthy.net,* accessed August 21, 2014, www.healthy.net/scr/article.aspx?Id=545.

13. Tufts Health & Nutrition Newsletter, eds., *Antioxidants* (Boston, Massachusetts: Tufts University, Gerald and Dorothy Friedman School of Nutrition Science and Policy) Pdf e-book, http://www.nutritionletter.tufts.edu/.

14. J.E. Enstrom, L.E. Kanim and M.A. Klein., "Vitamin C intake and mortality among a sample of the United States population," *Epidemiology* 3 no.3 (May 1992): 194-202, accessed August 21, 2014, http://www.ncbi.nlm.nih.gov/pubmed/1591317.

15 Tufts Health & Nutrition Newsletter, eds., *Antioxidants.*

16. John Matsen, ND, *Eating Alive: Prevention thru Good Digestion* (North Vancouver, British Columbia: Compton Books, 2002), 79.

17. Ross Pelton, RPh, and James B. LaValle, RPh, *The Nutritional Cost of Prescription Drugs: How to Maintain Good Nutrition While Using Prescription Drugs* (Englewood, Colorado: Morton Publishing Company, 2000).

18. *Orthomolecular Medicine, Orthomed.org,* accessed August 21, 2014, http://www.orthomed.org/.

19. Mark J. Bolland et al., "Vascular events in healthy older women receiving calcium supplementation: randomized controlled trial," *British Medical Journal* 336 no.7638 (2008): 262–266, accessed August 21, 2104, http://www.ncbi.nlm.nih.gov/pmc/articles/PMC2222999/.

20. A quality diet including cheese but not milk contains 700 mg of calcium per day. This is close to the 750 mg estimate stated in this article. "Food Rumors: Don't Bother Taking Calcium or Vitamin D," *Center for Research in the Public Interest, Nutrition Action Healthletter* (September 2012), 3.

21. Canada, Health Canada, "Daily Reference Intakes," last modified August 4, 2005, http://www.hc-sc.gc.ca/fn-an/nutrition/reference/table/ref_elements_tbl-eng.php.

22. Dr. Michael Schmidt, Dr. Lendon H. Sennet and Dr. Keith W. Sennet, *Beyond Antibiotics: 50 (or so) Ways to Boost Immunity and Avoid Antibiotics* (Berkeley, California: North Atlantic Books, 1993), 199.

23. Michelle Schoffro Cook, DNM, DAc, CNC, *The Ultimate pH Solution: Balance Your Body Chemistry to Prevent Disease and Lose Weight* (Toronto, Ontario: Harper Collins, 2008), 106.

24. "Some Calcium Supplements are Found to be Ineffective," *Newyorktimes.com,* (March 3, 1987) accessed September 10, 2014, .http://www.nytimes.com/1987/03/27/us/some-calcium-supplements-are-found-to-be-ineffective.html.

25. Michelle Schoffro Cook, *The Ultimate pH Solution,* 111.

26. Lyle MacWilliam, BSc, MSc, FP, *Comparative Guide to Nutritional Supplements,* 3rd edition (Vernon, British Columbia: Northern Dimensions Publishing, 2003).

27. Dr. Michael Schmidt, et al., *Beyond Antibiotics,* 199.

28. John Matsen, ND, *Eating Alive,* 10.

29. Dr. Bernard Jensen and Mark Anderson, *Empty Harvest: Understanding the Link between Our Food, Our Immunity, and Our Planet* (New York, New York: Penguin Putnam Inc., 1990), 148.

14: HEALTH BEGINS IN THE GUT

Death begins in the gut. ~ Nobel Prize winner Dr. Elie Metchnikoff, 1845–1916

Over one hundred years ago, Dr. Metchnikoff made his cryptic statement about gut health. Today, there is growing recognition of the link between the gut and overall health. In his 2013 book, *Clean Gut: The Breakthrough Plan for Eliminating the Root Cause of Disease and Revolutionizing Your Health,* Dr. Alejandro Junger makes the case that poor bowel function is at the root of most illness and disease.[1] Gut health refers to both the function and physical integrity of the intestinal tract. Many illnesses that start in the gut—irritable bowel, colitis, Crohn's—can lead to impaired immunity, hormone imbalances, and cardiovascular disease.

If death begins in the gut, health will also start there. In my clinical experience, a focus on my clients' gut health dramatically improves their health. One such client experienced dramatic results:

A.B. consulted with me soon after her doctor diagnosed her with Crohn's, an autoimmune bowel disease. Her doctor prescribed a steroid medication to control her symptoms: chronic diarrhea, abdominal bloating and pain, and weight loss. I started her on the anti-inflammatory diet and she improved. Over three years on this diet, and going through the healing protocol outlined in this chapter, she was able to go off the steroid medication without a return of Crohn's symptoms. She remains symptom free after eight years.

Unfortunately, few people in North America can boast good bowel function, at least not all the time. Restoring healthy function should be a primary focus of any attempt to restore health.

I have already stated, and it bears repeating, that the three responses that are critical to balanced body functioning are digestion, absorption, and elimination. These responses rely on several biochemical processes and organs. Enzymes, bile, and bacteria are all involved in digestion of food to allow absorption of nutrients the body needs. For example, dietary proteins must be broken down into their components, called amino acids. The vital organs—stomach, liver, gall bladder, pancreas, and small bowel—all have a role in digesting and absorbing nutrients from food. The large intestine and kidneys eliminate waste products. If you think of the digestive tract as a long river, it makes sense that problems *upstream* (stomach, liver, and pancreas) will worsen *downstream* and result in stress on the small and large intestines and the kidneys. The small intestines are the primary site for nutrient absorption; the large intestine and kidneys ensure efficient elimination of waste. When we do not absorb nutrients and eliminate waste, our health *will* suffer. This chapter focuses on how the gut loses its effectiveness, related symptoms, and how to restore healthy gut function.

Gut Biology

Dysbiosis is the term used to describe an imbalance in the constituents of the intestinal tract. This term originated with Dr. Elie Metchnikoff, who made the dramatic statement "death begins the gut." He was awarded the Nobel Prize in 1908 for his discovery that friendly bacterial flora is essential to the absorption of nutrients from food. The origins of the term dysbiosis come from *dys*, meaning incorrect, and *biosis*, meaning life. Its opposite, *symbiosis*, means to reside together harmoniously. *Dysbiosis* is therefore a lack of harmony or balance that will pose a threat to health.

Dysbiosis is an intestinal imbalance in which harmful organisms have taken over as the dominant species. To appreciate how this imbalance develops, it is important to understand gut biology. The lower part of the small intestine and the colon contain microbes, mostly bacteria, working in a mutually beneficial relationship with each other and with us. These microbes include three components: beneficial bacteria (e.g., *lactobacillus acidophilus*), commensal bacteria (e.g. *E. coli* and *streptococci*), and pathogenic organisms (bacteria, viruses, and parasites). Pathogens are normally low in numbers, unless there is a depletion of the other two components—beneficial and commensal bacteria. When the pathogenic constituents overpopulate the gut flora, a dysbiosis occurs.

If not corrected, a dysbiosis will weaken the function of the intestinal tract, resulting in malabsorption of nutrients and poor elimination of toxins. Few people realize how important healthy gut flora is to immune system function. If not corrected, a dysbiosis can either suppress immunity or make it hyper-reactive, a state that can trigger an autoimmune disease. In my clinical experience, dysbiosis can take years to develop and typically results from a combination of unhealthy choices, medication side effects, and/or infections—one or more of the following:

- Overeating and/or irregular eating patterns
- Eating foods to which you are sensitive or intolerant
- Eating too much processed food (additives and low nutrient content)
- Overconsumption of sugar, including alcohol (sugar feeds mold/fungi in the gut)
- Overexposure to antibiotics which kill off all gut microbes indiscriminately, both good and bad varieties. Sources include antibiotic medication and meat contaminated with antibiotics
- Drinking chlorinated water
- Bacterial infections from food, contaminated drinking water, and international travel
- Parasites, waterborne, e.g., *Giardia lamblia* or *cryptosporidium*
- Parasites from pets can expose us to 240 infectious diseases
- Parasites from wildlife, e.g., Lyme disease from deer ticks

Dysbiosis involves three types of imbalances: overpopulation by harmful bacteria, overgrowth of mold/fungi, and parasitic infections. Harmful bacteria typically involve acute gastrointestinal upset (diarrhea) that is usually short-lived. Fungal overgrowth and parasitic infections can become chronic conditions. Identifying these issues can be tricky because of the vagueness and variety of symptoms, and because it is a functional problem, rather than a physical one. A functional imbalance will not show up in medical tests such as X-rays, ultrasounds, or colonoscopies all of which identify only physical issues. The most reliable indicators of dysbiosis are symptoms, which vary from person to person. Not all the symptoms listed below need be present to conclude that this imbalance exists. Naturopath Dr. John Matsen, well known for his insights on dysbiosis, believes this condition to be widespread. He states, "Nearly everyone's intestinal flora is imbalanced and overgrown with the 'bad guys.'"[2]

Bacterial or Fungal Overgrowth

There are several symptoms associated with these conditions. My clinical experience is that four or five of the listed symptoms must be present to suspect this overgrowth:

Abdominal bloating and cramps

Intestinal gas—candida gives off neurotoxins, acids, aldehydes, and gases

Irregular bowels—chronic diarrhea

Allergies or sinusitis

Cravings for sweets or starches—they feed mold/fungi

Tongue coated

Low energy, apathetic

Anxiety—unexplained

Poor concentration or "brain fog"

Hyperactivity in children

Recurrent bladder and vaginal infections

Skin—eczema, rashes, acne

Toenail fungus or athlete's foot

Prostate issues (male)

In the holistic health field, a fungal overgrowth (often referred to as candidiasis) is very common, yet often goes undetected. In the *Complete Candida Yeast Guidebook,* Jeanne Marie Martin and Zoltan Rona, MD tell us candida an underlying factor in several conditions, including chronic fatigue syndrome, chronic allergies, fibromyalgia, premenstrual syndrome, endometriosis, vaginal infections, and bladder infections.[3]

Parasitic Infections

Symptoms of parasitic infections vary widely, perhaps because there are numerous types (e.g., roundworms, pinworms, hookworms, and protozoans.) My experience is that several, but not all, of the following symptoms must exist to consider parasites as the culprit:

Abdominal bloating and gas

Excess belching or burping

Irregular bowels—constipation and/or loose stools or diarrhea

Anemia, pale or weak

Fatigue, unexplained

Loss of appetite or hungry soon after eating

Nausea

Bedwetting (in children)

Recently developed food sensitivities

Teeth grinding

Drool while sleeping

Disturbed sleep

Dry lips

White spots on nails

Itchy inside the ears

Irritability

Poor memory or foggy thinking

Besides symptoms, it is critical to consider life events, current health status, and health history to assess the potential for parasitic infections. I always ask my clients about travelling to countries with different climates and foods. Typical questions are "When travelling, did you experience gastrointestinal illness?" and "After this trip, did your health return to its previous state or are there lingering issues such as low energy and poor digestion?" When clients answer "yes" to these questions *and* they have several of the above symptoms, I *always* find that an anti-parasitic protocol makes dramatic improvements in how they feel, in particular if they have a history of irritable bowel or colitis.

In Chapter 5, I discuss the health costs of long-term parasitic infections and their role in bowel disease (colitis, Crohn's disease), chronic fatigue syndrome, hypoglycemia, ulcers, and arthritis. Because parasites rob the body of essential nutrients, they eventually impair the immune system. Naturopath, author, and practitioner of alternative medicine, Dr. Huldah Clark linked chronic parasitic infections to cancer and many other illnesses.[4] People can suffer with unrecognized chronic infections because of some poorly understood aspects of parasites.

- Parasitic infections are more common than people think. Government health organizations estimate that 40 percent of the population has, or has had, a parasitic infection.

- Parasites come from several sources: water, food, sexual contact, animals, and insects such as mosquitos and sandflies.

- Parasites are not immediately life threatening because their goal is to live with us, not kill us off.

- Parasites do not limit themselves to the digestive tract. Nutritionist and author Ann Louise Gittleman emphasizes parasites can damage almost any organ or body system: the liver, brain, lungs, uterus, and joints..

- Because Western medicine views such infections as a tropical medicine issue, testing is often not even considered. Some of my clients must beg their doctors for parasitic testing.

- Parasites are very good at not making themselves known. Testing can easily miss them. My clinical and personal experience bears this out.

    When she was 12 years old, my daughter contracted an amoeba-type parasite, *blastocystis hominus*. Although the medical doctor did not consider this parasite pathogenic, it took four years to eliminate. Initial medical testing for parasites was negative. It took another two years through consultation with alternative health practitioners to detect the parasitic infection. A specialized lab in the United States identified the amoeba. Even after this was known, the medical treatments were not effective. After years of entrenchment by the parasite, her immune system was depressed. It took extra therapeutic measures to eliminate the parasite and restore good health, which she now enjoys.

In my clinical practice, I have had several clients who, like my daughter, had suffered for years with parasitic-type symptoms. Sometimes, medical doctors do not consider testing for parasites. After an anti-parasitic protocol, these clients reported significant improvement in their bowel function and overall health.

"Leaky Gut"

If a dysbiosis, whether from fungal overgrowth or parasites, is not addressed, physical damage to the intestinal tract will eventually result, specifically to the microvilli in the intestinal wall. This leads to increased permeability, a state in which food particles do not digest properly before they try to pass through the intestinal wall. In holistic health practice, this is referred to as *leaky gut*. The immune system reacts to the undigested food particles as if they were invaders, and this triggers allergies and even autoimmune disorders such as Crohn's. My view is that a diagnosis of colitis (inflammation of the colon) is a sign of leaky gut, which therapeutic diets and cleansing protocols can remedy.

Caution: I do not recommend self-administration of cleansing protocols. My purpose here is to raise awareness of their value and to help you determine if you would benefit from one. The need for cleansing protocols should always be determined, and their administration supervised by a holistic health practitioner.

Cleansing Protocols

The selection of a cleansing protocol will depend on the type of dysbiosis—either mold/fungi or parasitic. There is often an assortment of intestinal "critters."

An overgrowth of mold and fungi provides a welcoming environment for parasites, so both types of dysbiosis often go hand in hand. Intestinal cleansing protocols may be needed for both types of dysbiosis, but in separate protocols and at different times.

Systemic cleansing may be required to address imbalances that have moved outside the digestive tract in the bloodstream and tissues. Symptoms of systemic imbalances include fingernail or toenail fungus, yeast infections (vaginal), persistent fatigue, and lack of concentration or brain fog. These issues are indicators that the immune system has been overwhelmed by an intestinal dysbiosis, thus allowing mold and fungus to spread through the body. Some of my clients go through both digestive and systemic cleansing before they feel well again.

Preparation for Cleansing

The first step in restoring healthy gut flora and bowel function is to ensure that both foods and environment are health supportive. Jumping right into cleansing will be counterproductive, and the condition will certainly persist. This happens often with those who self-administer cleanses. These are my recommended steps before starting a cleanse protocol:

- Follow the Quality Diet outlined in Chapter 7.
- Eat the right diet for you, including avoidance of foods and additives to which you are sensitive. See Chapter 8.
- Have foods high in prebiotics, i.e., factors that promote healthy gut flora. Inulin is a compound that contains prebiotics. It is found in vegetables such as artichokes, garlic, leeks, onions, and chicory; grains such as oats; seeds such as flax; and fermented soy, such as miso or tempeh.
- Avoid wheat, wheat bran, and corn. These grains are difficult to digest. It is okay to have small amounts of rice, millet, and quinoa.
- Ideal proteins: Fish, free-range chicken, and eggs.
- If dairy is tolerated, have organic plain yogurt and kefir.
- Pumpkin seeds, garlic, and onions are all antifungal, antibacterial, and anti-parasitic.
- Avoid sugar, e.g., white sugar, and alcohol. This includes not adding sugar to foods and avoiding foods with added sugar, such as fruit juices, fruit drinks, and yogurt. It also means limiting fruit to only two per day.
- Avoid foods that tend to mold: refrigerated food, peanuts, grapes, strawberries, and melons.
- Avoid mushrooms, which are fungi.
- Avoid foods high in starches, such as potatoes—eat only one to two servings weekly.
- Avoid yeasted bread—use sourdough bread, which is easier to digest.
- Drink lots of water, ideally filtered of contaminants.

- Drink supportive herbal teas: rooibos, peppermint, ginger.
- Avoid stimulants—chocolate and caffeinated drinks.

If there is little change in symptoms after following these recommendations, a cleanse protocol will be required to restore a healthy gut flora.

Cleansing Agents

During a cleanse protocol, the above preparation diet continues. There are three types of cleanse supplements: herbal, elimination support, and probiotics. Herbal cleansing formulas for mold and fungi typically include one or more of the following: barberry root extract, echinacea, garlic, grapefruit seed extract, goldenseal, Oregon grape, or pau d'arco. Formulas specific to parasites include some combination of black walnut, cloves, pumpkin, quassia, sweet wormwood, and yarrow. Elimination support is critical to ensure the release of toxins from the "die off" of yeast or parasites. This support includes ingredients with different roles. Dandelion, beet, and parsley help the liver fulfill its role in handling toxins that are released during cleansing. To ensure the bowels move regularly, one or more of the following may be needed: cascara sagrada, senna, magnesium, psyllium, and inulin. Bentonite clay is also beneficial to mop up toxins and ensure elimination. The third type of cleanse supplement is a probiotic. Herbal cleansing agents reduce *all* bacteria in the gut, even the beneficial kind. Since digestion and immunity both benefit from probiotics, their depletion must be avoided to ensure the success of the cleanse. Some people with weak digestion may also need a digestive enzyme during cleansing. In more severe cases, I recommend general nutritional support, such as a "greens" supplements and vitamins C and D to help the body stay strong.

The specific protocol depends on the number and severity of the symptoms and estimated duration of the condition. Based on the assessment of these issues, a holistic health practitioner selects the appropriate supplement formulas, dosage, and duration of the protocol. If dosages are too low, or if the protocol is stopped too soon, the condition will reoccur. With long-standing dysbiosis, I find cleansing can take three months or more. Fungal overgrowth and parasites are often both present, which requires an antifungal protocol, followed by an anti-parasitic one. Because of the life cycles of parasites (egg, larva, and adult), cleansing must continue until all life cycles are addressed. If symptoms suggest a systemic cleanse is needed, cleansing may include periodic changes in the cleanse agent.

My clients who complete cleansing protocols report dramatic improvements in health. They are often amazed to have increased energy, improved digestion, normalized bowel function, and relief from allergy symptoms. Often sensitivities to food are also reduced.

What to expect during cleansing

People can be discouraged from going through a cleanse protocol because of some unpleasant but natural reactions, also called healing reactions (see Chapter 10).

For cleansing to be effective, some symptoms may become temporarily worse. Protocols that cleanse the intestinal tract represent a challenge to the intestinal status quo, which may have existed for some time. In effect, the intestinal tract becomes a battleground in which cleanse agents are duking it out with harmful microbes. Consider a situation in which you have food poisoning; there is vomiting and perhaps diarrhea, which, while unpleasant, are necessary to eliminate the bacteria and restore healthy balance. As explained in Chapter 5, we may be overloaded with food chemicals, pharmaceuticals, as well as infectious agents that cleansing will release. Parasites release toxins during their die-off, which can produce cramping, gas, irregularity, and even flu-like symptoms.

Reactions may also go in cycles; some days, there will be renewed energy, while other days, the old symptoms can return. The overall health status of the individuals also plays a role in the severity of reactions. As long as symptoms can be tolerated, the protocol should continue. In cleansing, it is critical not to misinterpret symptoms and conclude that it is making things worse. What can be perceived as a negative reaction should be celebrated as a sign that an imbalance is being corrected.

Common cleanse symptoms and their reasons:

Mild headaches are typically the result of toxins release faster than the liver—our main organ of detoxification—can handle. Often my clients experience headaches during the first week of cleansing.

Constipation can be a sign of excess toxins in the lower intestinal tract that the body cannot eliminate fast enough. If this happens, more support for elimination is needed. However, low water intake could also be the cause.

Loose stools are common because some cleanse supplements encourage bowel movements. It is more beneficial to be on the loose side to ensure elimination of the microbes that are killed during cleansing.

Skin rashes are not a good sign, as this is an indicator of poor elimination through the bowels and urinary tract. Toxins are trying to exit through the skin instead.

Fatigue is the most common cleanse symptom reported by my clients. Cleansing asks the body to do extra work, which can leave less energy for other activities.

Adverse symptoms should last no longer than a week after starting a cleanse. During this time, it is important to rest and avoid excess exercise. Unless symptoms are unbearable, it is important to keep going. Stopping a cleanse prematurely can cause reoccurrence of health concerns, often after a short time period. If symptoms continue for longer than a few weeks, this is a sign of more serious health issues that require medical attention.

I cannot emphasize enough the health risks associated with a dysbiosis that is not addressed. Putting up with this imbalance or medicating its symptoms will worsen the condition and, in my experience, increase the risk of damage in the intestinal tract, bowel disease, and impaired immunity.

Repair the Gut

After cleansing is completed, the intestinal wall will need repair, in particular if there have been symptoms of leaky gut, such as bowel disorders or allergies. The need for repair will also depend on how long the dysbiosis existed prior to the cleanse. A repair protocol can include one or more of the following:

Anti-Inflammatory Diet (Appendix 4)

Antioxidants, such as vitamins C and E

Amino acids, L-glutamine and lysine, or the organo-sulphur compound *Methylsulfonylmethane* (MSM)

Herbs, such as slippery elm and marshmallow root

Enzymes with bromelain and papain

Probiotic

A holistic nutritionist or other holistic health practitioner best determines the specifics and duration of a repair protocol. Because of individual weaknesses, dysbiosis can recur more easily in the presence of a chronic intestinal condition or repeated use of antibiotics. For some, cleansing may be needed on a yearly or more frequent basis. A return of symptoms is the best indicator of the need to cleanse again.

Chapter Notes

1. Alejandro Junger, MD, *Clean Gut: The Breakthrough Plan for Eliminating the Root Cause of Disease and Revolutionizing Your Health* (New York: HarperOne, 2013).

2. John Matsen, ND, *Eating Alive: Prevention thru Good Digestion* (North Vancouver, British Columbia: Compton Books, 2002), 31.

3. Jeanne Marie Martin with Zoltan P. Rona, MD, *Complete Candida Yeast Guidebook: Everything You Need to Know About Prevention, Treatment & Diet.,* Revised 2nd edition (Roseville, California: Prima Publishing, 2000), 25.

4. Hulda Regeher Clark, PhD, ND, *The Prevention of All Cancers* (Chula Vista, California: New Century Press, 2007).

15: GET THE LEAD OUT

Many of the diseases that baffle our physicians (often called the "diseases of aging" or "diseases of civilization") are the result of toxic overload. ~ Raymond Francis[1]

In Chapters 1, 2 and 5, I outline the likelihood of our exposure to toxins from several sources—air, water, food production, food processing, food packaging, radiation, and electromagnetic frequencies. There are serious health risks related to overexposure to naturally occurring heavy metals (e.g., aluminum, lead, mercury), synthetic chemicals (e.g., pesticides, herbicides, plastics), and even food additives. The degree to which health is affected depends on two factors: the extent of exposure and the individual's ability to eliminate toxins from the body. It may not be possible to avoid all toxins, even by adhering to the recommendations in Chapter 7: Quality Food and Toxin-Free Living. The EXtension TOXicology NETwork, a cooperative effort of several universities in the United States, explains our challenges in this statement: "The possible toxic effects of exposure to a particular chemical depend on many factors. These include the characteristics of the chemical and the individual exposed…Unfortunately scientists have not been able to determine exactly how each of these factors will affect any specific individual."[2]

In my clinical experience, some people become toxic because they do not eliminate them effectively. They are what I call *poor eliminators*, and often they are not aware of this metabolic weakness. I can estimate who is a poor eliminator and their extent of toxic overload based on health history, nutritional symptomatology, and through the Bioenergetic Evaluation. Poor toxin elimination is more common with older individuals but can be an issue at any age. A 12-year-old client showed little improvement in her health issues until she completed a detoxification protocol, often referred to simply as "detox."

A detox is a therapeutic protocol that is best administered and supervised by a holistic health practitioner. For this reason, I debated whether to include detoxing in this book, but I elected to do so because there is growing awareness of the value of detoxing; it has become trendy with increasing availability of "detox kits" in health stores. Detoxing is also a label used to describe some weight-loss programs. However, self-administered detox programs may not address your specific issues and, as a result, will not detoxify *your* body effectively. Because of the complicated nature of detoxing, the do-it-yourself approach could even cause undesirable effects. Perhaps this is why there is also some bad press about detoxification protocols. This chapter outlines the signs of poor elimination and toxic overload, provides a toxicity prevention protocol, and explains the detoxification process. With this information, you can assess the various detox options and make a choice that will best serve your needs.

The information in this chapter is for general information. To determine your need for a detoxification protocol, I recommend consultation with a holistic health practitioner with expertise in such protocols.

The Detox Debate

You might well ask, if detoxing is so beneficial, why is so little attention paid to it by the medical system? The answer is simple; those who have the ear of the medical system downplay the need for a detox protocol. In *An Apple a Day: The Myths, Misconceptions, and Truths about the Foods We Eat,* chemist and university professor, Joe Schwarcz, states: "Our bodies are engaged in detoxification all the time. Our liver and kidneys are very adept at removing undesirable intruders."[3] In Chapter 5, I present evidence that toxins in our environment are adversely affecting our health. Many government bodies and organizations are alerting us to the risks of toxic exposure. This begs the question: If we are eliminating toxins so well, why are toxins such a threat to our health?

At the crux of the debate about the need for detox protocols is the body's ability to eliminate waste. I have known people who have smoked all their lives and maintain good health; these are no doubt efficient eliminators. However, a woman I know developed lung cancer, even though she neither smoked nor was she exposed to second-hand smoke. I suspect she was a poor eliminator. There are several reasons we can become poor eliminators, such as inherited weakness, a low-quality diet, a chronic condition, or a past illness. Chapter 10 explains how it can take several stressors to upset healthy balance and leave us vulnerable to illness. If toxins accumulate beyond the body's ability to eliminate, there will be negative effects on health. Because toxins can accumulate anywhere in the body—in tissues, joints, organs, or blood vessels—health may suffer in a variety of ways that are discussed in Chapter 5. If there is no action to eliminate the toxins, health will continue to decline. A detoxification protocol becomes an absolute necessity.

Understanding the Body's Detoxification System

The liver has the primary role in eliminating toxins with help from several organs and systems that serve as elimination pathways. These include the intestinal tract, urinary tract, lymph system, respiratory tract, blood, and skin. If wastes and toxins are not excreted through one or more of these pathways, the liver's ability to detoxify is challenged. Toxic overload ensues and health will be adversely affected. The good news is that there are bodily symptoms of poor elimination that precede toxic overload. In Chapter 11, I promote the understanding of bodily symptoms as important signals that we should not ignore or medicate away. Here, we consider symptoms specifically to help you determine if you are at risk of toxicity.

The type of symptoms that present themselves helps determine the extent and severity of poor elimination. The intestinal and urinary tracts are the primary and preferred pathways of elimination, making them the first to be affected. A compromised intestinal system displays one or more of these symptoms: constipation, irregularity, breakouts around the chin, and headaches. Urinary congestion produces frequent or urgent urination, puffy eyes, low back pain, or stiff joints. Once these pathways are compromised, the other less preferred ones are called upon to assist. This means that symptoms related to respiration, the lymph system and skin, point to more severe elimination problems and a higher risk of toxicity.

Lymph congestion presents as one or more of these symptoms: fatigue, swollen ankles, hard bumps under the skin, frequent illness, and skin tags. Symptoms of stress in respiratory elimination include shortness of breath, lightheadedness, fatigue, tendency to chest colds, and asthma. In holistic health practice, we consider the issue underlying asthma to be poor elimination through the intestinal tract. Treating the breathing problems associated with asthma will not address the underlying poor elimination. Consider a scenario in which firefighters tend to a building on fire with smoke pouring out of every window. If the fire fighters spray water only on the smoke, they will not put out the fire. Their focus would be on the symptom (smoke) rather than the fire itself (the root cause). Likewise, there are symptoms of toxicity in the body we can ease with medication, but this leaves unseen toxins to damage our bodies from within.

Elimination through the skin is the least preferred of the body's pathways. Some toxins are eliminated via the skin through sweat, which explains the benefit of saunas and exercise that induces sweating. However, excess excretion of toxins through the skin signals a breakdown in one or more of the preferred pathways: intestinal, urinary, and respiratory. Toxins passing through the skin may present as rashes, itching, acne, boils, and eczema. Rather than recognizing these symptoms as warning signs of poor elimination, the medical approach is typically treatment with creams and salves. But skin problems are a critical sign of the need for detoxification. Masking symptoms of toxin release through the skin becomes in itself a threat to health.

Preventing Toxicity

It is possible to avoid toxic accumulation by following the recommendations in Chapter 7: Quality Food and Toxin-Free Living. But, if you are continually exposed to toxins (e.g., air pollution, work environments) or you are a poor eliminator (see symptoms above), a quality diet may not be enough to prevent toxic overload, and you will suffer adverse health effects.

I recommend periodic use of a gentle and easy-to-follow detoxification protocol. It has great preventative benefit when followed for three to seven days and repeated seasonally. With higher or prolonged toxic exposure, I recommend the seven-day application repeated monthly. This protocol is not appropriate for those with chronic illness (e.g., cancer, cardiovascular disease, diabetes, ulcers, or autoimmune disease) unless there is supervision by a holistic health practitioner.

The **gentle detoxification protocol** has three elements:

a) **On rising in the morning,** drink a glass of spring or filtered water with juice squeezed from half a lemon, plus a pinch of ground ginger, and a dash of cayenne pepper.

b) **During the morning ingest *only* whole fruit and vegetables/vegetables juices.** This eases any stress on digestion and supports healthy elimination. The concept of having only fruit and vegetables in the morning is central to the *Fit for Life* program of the 1980s, except that it was espoused as a daily health regimen.[4] Ideal fruits are ones that are not too sweet, such as apples, pears, peaches, blueberries. Ideal vegetables are green, dark green leafy, and orange vegetables, either raw, juiced, or in soups. Also include foods that support detoxification, such as beets, garlic and onion.

c) **For the rest of the day**, eat whole foods recommended in Chapter 7, including these food groups: proteins (animal or vegetable), fats, grains, and vegetables. No additional fruit is recommended because all the daily servings are consumed in the morning.

The gentle detox can be followed for up to seven days and repeated monthly. When followed for at least three days consecutively, this protocol will trigger the body to release toxins. To ensure their elimination, the liver and intestinal tract will need support. This is more important if there are already symptoms of liver stress or an intestinal imbalance, as outlined in Chapter 11. Detox supports include some combination of herbs such as milk thistle, dandelion extract, and/or dandelion root tea. Fibre is also essential to help eliminate toxins. I recommend fibre from inulin (artichokes, garlic, leeks, onions, and chicory), and ground flax. It is also advisable to avoid stimulants such as caffeine and alcohol. Rest and moderate exercise also support healing.

Prevention is the primary purpose of the gentle detoxification protocol, but I have also used it in three other ways:

Support during weight loss

Toxins are often stored in body fat. As a result, loss of body fat can be accompanied by the release of toxins into circulation. The gentle detox alleviates unwanted symptoms from toxin release.

After known exposure to toxins from:

Prolonged adherence to low-quality diet

Ongoing exposure through the workplace

Removal of mercury amalgam fillings

Proximity to pesticide spraying

As an indicator of toxic overload

If after three days on this protocol, there are unpleasant symptoms such as headaches, fatigue, or light-headedness, I would assess the need for a therapeutic detox protocol.

How to Assess Toxicity

Based on the number of toxins in our environment, almost everyone will benefit from detoxification support. Unfortunately, no medical tests can identify toxicity. Some holistic health practitioners use hair analysis to test for heavy metals, but its reliability has been questioned because of great variations in the results from different labs.[5] I rely on two factors to determine toxicity: history of exposure and symptoms. You can assess your exposure risk from the information in Chapter 5. because of the potential for exposure in North America, I believe most of us have accumulated *some* toxins in our bodies. Symptoms are highly reliable indicators that toxicity is at a level that warrants a detoxification protocol. Symptoms vary and can affect any body system, including:

- Digestive—constipation, diarrhea, nausea, heartburn, bloating, colic, metallic taste in mouth
- Circulatory/vascular—shortness of breath, rapid heartbeat, chest pain, water retention, headache)
- Nervous—poor concentration, failing memory, anxiety, irritability, learning disabilities
- Muscular—muscle twitches or tremors, heavy feeling in arms and legs
- Immune—sinus problems, lung congestion, frequent illness
- Skin—hives, rashes, itching, skin tags, sallow complexion, dry mucous membranes
- Hormonal—infertility, impotence
- Unspecified system—unexplained fatigue, weight loss, hair loss

Because there are varied symptoms of toxicity, they can easily be misinterpreted as other health issues, including the flu, allergic reactions, or even as natural signs of aging. Some people blame their heredity and take this fatalistic view such as "my mother had this [illness, condition], so I do too." A holistic assessment of toxicity symptoms must consider duration, frequency, and severity.

Detoxification Prerequisites

Consider detoxification as an advanced course in college or university. There are prerequisite *courses* to go through. These courses or steps include a health-supportive diet, cleansing the digestive tract, and drainage of elimination organs (liver, kidneys). People often tell me they tried detoxing, and it did not work. Often they had not prepared for the detox by first changing their diet and supporting their elimination pathways. They did not honour the natural healing process.

Always Start with Diet

All healing starts with the right dietary foundation—eat quality foods (Chapter 7) and eat your right diet (Chapter 8). Using food for healing (Chapter 12) may also help ensure that the body's detoxification function is restored.

Cleansing

Before a detoxification protocol, the digestive pathways of elimination must be functioning well. This is accomplished through cleansing of the intestinal tract (Chapter 14) and drainage of the liver and kidneys. Skipping the "required course" of cleansing and going directly to detoxification can both negate the benefit of the detox and cause undue suffering, such as headaches, intestinal upsets, fatigue, and flu-like symptoms.

Drainage

Many people have heard about detoxification. Few have heard of drainage—a critical function of the liver and kidneys. When toxins enter the body (or release from tissues), they first go through the bloodstream before passing through the liver and kidneys for elimination. During a detox, when there is an extra load of toxins, these organs must be functioning optimally. If these organs are already stressed, toxins may not be eliminated at all, but recirculated and stored elsewhere in the body. My clinical experience has borne this out—clients with poor drainage who attempt a detox protocol will experience unbearable symptoms and be discouraged from continuing. It is therefore critical to understand the symptoms that denote poor drainage.

Since drainage is primarily the job of the liver and kidneys, symptoms of stress in these organs point to the need for a drainage protocol. Symptoms of liver and kidney stress are discussed in Chapter 11. A holistic health practitioner can help determine if the liver and kidneys require drainage that includes eating the right diet for individual needs, consuming adequate fibre, and the therapeutic use of herbs and/or homeopathic remedies.

Detoxification Process

Detoxification protocols release toxins from anywhere they are stored in the body, and it can be anywhere. In a self-protective way, an overburdened liver may have stored toxins where they would not cause immediate harm. Think of it like this: You have too little time to clean up for important company. Instead of putting all the clutter away in its rightful place, you throw it in a closet, so it is out of sight. The liver does this, too. The membranes of the large intestine are a primary storage place for toxins.[6] Once toxins line the walls of the intestines, effective elimination of waste (toxins) is further compromised, which can lead to further toxic overload. Fat cells are another one of the liver's favored storage places for toxins. As noted earlier in this chapter, losing weight can release toxins that have been stored in fat cells and result in unpleasant reactions. Such reactions are identified in the next section, "What to Expect during Detoxification." Other possible storage places for toxins include joints, reproductive organs, and skin. Conditions related to these systems—arthritis, endometriosis, fibroids, skin conditions—are often related to accumulated toxins.

To be effective and safe, detoxification protocols use diet and supplements that both release *and* remove toxins. Certain supplements focus on the release of toxins from where they are stored (fat tissues, joints, nerve endings, blood vessels), while others eliminate them. The protocol must consider the health status of the individual and be supervised by a holistic health practitioner—holistic nutritionist, naturopath or homeopath.

What to Expect during Detoxification

We can liken a detox protocol to spring-cleaning a house. We pull things out of their usual places, stir up dust, and create general disarray. The same thing happens during detoxification of the body. The protocol's intent is to take toxins out of the tissues where they have been stored and release them into circulation through the bloodstream. If toxins are not readily eliminated, they will re-circulate in the body and cause unwanted symptoms, such as headaches, foggy thinking, poor concentration, and bowel irregularity. These cleanse symptoms are natural, but they should be short-lived and tolerable. If unwanted symptoms continue past the first week of the detox or they are not tolerable, it is because there is poor drainage through the liver and/or kidneys or poor function in elimination pathways—intestines, lymph, respiration (see previous section on Cleansing and Drainage).

If unwanted symptoms are not tolerable, one or more actions may be necessary: stop the detox for a few days; stop the detox and undergo cleansing and/or drainage; continue to detox but add more support for elimination through diet or supplementation; reduce the dosage of detox agents. This is when the expertise of the holistic health practitioner is needed to select the course of action that provides the intended benefit from a detox protocol. Medicating away detox symptoms (e.g., taking a pain reliever) will only interfere with the detoxification process, perhaps negate its effectiveness. I always advise my clients not to fear symptoms the body produces during a detox. While side effects from medical drugs can be threats to health, unpleasant reactions from a detox are usually signs that a harmful agent is being released from the body. If you feel no different in the first week of a detox, you should question the need for the protocol.

A detox can be one of the longest protocols to complete successfully. It can take several months and may have to be repeated on an annual or semi-annual basis. Duration and frequency of detox protocols will depend on continued exposure to toxins and the individual's ability to eliminate toxins.

In summary, detoxification is a high-level therapeutic protocol that can have unintended effects if the required steps are not followed or the essential therapeutic agents and supports are not present. For this reason, I do not provide a specific detoxification protocol to follow here. My aim is to provide an understanding of detox protocols so that you seek the best possible advice for your needs. Detoxes must always be geared to the individual's health status and level of toxicity, and this should be determined and supervised by a holistic health practitioner.

Chapter Notes

1. Raymond Francis, MSc, *Never Be Sick Again: Health is a Choice, Learn How to Choose it* (Deerfield Beach, Florida: Health Communications, 2002), 146.

2. "Toxicology Information Briefs," *The EXtension TOXicology NETwork, University of California-Davis, Oregon State University, Michigan State University, Cornell University, and the University of Idaho, Extoxnet.orst.edu*, accessed March 2014, http://extoxnet.orst.edu/.

3. Joe Schwarcz, PhD, *An Apple a Day: The Myths, Misconceptions, and Truths About the Foods We Eat* (Toronto, Ontario: HarperCollins, 2007), 344.

4. Harvey Diamond and Marilyn Diamond, *Fit for Life II: Living Health* (New York (New York: Warner Books, 1987).

5. Sun Namkoong, et al., "Reliability on Intra-Laboratory and Inter-Laboratory Data of Hair Mineral Analysis Comparing with Blood Analysis," *Annals of Dermatology* 25 no.1 (Feb 2013): 67–72, accessed September 20, 2014, http://www.ncbi.nlm.nih.gov/pmc/articles/PMC3582931/.

6. John Matsen, ND, *Eating Alive: Prevention thru Good Digestion* (North Vancouver, British Columbia: Compton Books, 2002), 147.

YOUR HOLISTIC GUIDE TO BEING WELL

I believe we all have the capacity to *be well* as I have defined it: living without undue concern, or medication needed, for a health issue or emotional problem. Unfortunately, in the 21st century with all the threats to our health, it is all too common for us to be *un*well. There is an increasing incidence of health conditions—asthma, allergies, overweight, and digestive disorders—that, while not immediately life threatening, are warning signs of poor health down the road. We need not resign ourselves to living with these conditions or the suffering they cause. We can also avoid the realization of gloomy predictions about the state of health in North America. A 2013 report by the Heart and Stroke Foundation of Canada predicts "a 10-year gap between how long we live, and how long we live in health."[1] This dire warning means that, for most of us, old age will mean ill health. The report cites lifestyle choices such as poor diet, sedentary living, undue stress, smoking, and excess alcohol consumption as the primary reasons for aging in poor health. The message is clear: healthy nutrition and lifestyle can put us firmly on the path to wellness. To begin this journey, we need to be aware of our choices and attitudes, and change those that are not health supportive. If we become active participants in our own health care, we can be well now, and for longer than statistics might predict.

In this book, I outline how everyone can be well through a holistic health approach. This is not a theory; the evidence is abundant. Epigenetics research has established that even with genetic predispositions to certain conditions, we are not doomed to developing them. Good nutrition and emotional balance can suppress the genes that can trigger illness and disease. To paraphrase Hippocrates, we *can* let food be our medicine. We must also stop defining our health care only as treating illness and fixing body parts. Waiting until we are ill to make health-promoting changes is not the answer. Taking medications to suppress symptoms can mask health issues and stop the search for their underlying causes. Some in the medical community call the Western medical approach "sick care." This approach does little to help us be well.

My Holistic Model of Wellness illustrates how much control we *can* have over our health. Depending on our choices—nutrition, physical and social environment, and movement—we can either support or challenge our health. Still, healthy choices are not clear-cut. In North America, food quality and conflicting dietary advice can make it difficult to make health-promoting choices. The definition of a healthy diet is subject to political influence. Flaws in nutrition research and myths about certain foods add to the confusion about what to eat. There are real and present threats from toxins, both natural and man-made. Emotions, thought patterns, and beliefs can have negative effects on physical health. In response to these challenges, I present comprehensive holistic guides for diet, lifestyle, and the emotional state that promotes being well.

Being well is not just about our choices; our response to diet and environment also play a role. We are biochemically unique; we respond in our own ways and therefore need an individualized approach. The Holistic Model of Wellness is unique among health models because it allows for individual differences in how we respond to foods and environmental factors. Rather than provide a prescriptive plan for diet and lifestyle, I describe how to find the diet that is right for individual needs and how to identify habits, emotions, and beliefs that upset emotional balance.

Through a holistic health approach, you can be well now *and* prevent illness down the road. At the point when the body malfunctions, symptoms reliably show there is a loss of balance, a loss of homeostasis. Instead of the mainstream focus on medicating symptoms, a holistic approach uses symptoms as warning signs that point us to healing steps that prevent illness. Restoring healthy balance holistically works because it taps into the body's natural healing processes.

For any health imbalance, diet change is the first step. Healing diets and the way we eat food have tremendous power to support the body's natural healing processes. Nutritional supplements have an important role, but should be considered as an adjunct to healing, not a replacement for dietary change. Therapeutic protocols of cleansing and detoxification can make a big difference to health outcomes, but should not be attempted without practitioner supervision.

You *can* be well *if* you think and act holistically about your health care. It is imperative to take personal responsibility, be proactive about your choices, and attend to your body's signals. If there are symptoms of concern and a medical doctor has ruled out illness, it is critical to continue searching for answers using a holistic approach.

In summary, I offer ten guidelines that epitomize my holistic health approach for being well:

1. Give your body quality fuel—food and fluids
2. Avoid toxins in food, water, and the environment
3. Eat the right diet for your needs—rule out food sensitivities and intolerances
4. Seek emotional balance, whatever your situation
5. Use the body's natural healing powers—avoid quick-fix remedies
6. Exercise regularly at a moderate level
7. Understand what bodily symptoms mean about the root causes of health issues
8. Use healing diets and foods with specific healing properties
9. Use supplements in ways that aid healing, rather than for symptom relief

10. Recognize the symptoms that point to the need for therapeutic protocols and consult with a holistic health practitioner

After reading this book, you should have a sense of which guidelines require more change for you personally. Some changes will be more challenging. In particular, "seeking emotional balance," for most of us, involves lifelong study and practice. It is for this reason that my focus is not on ensuring emotional balance, because no one is perfectly balanced in this area. However, the journey is as important as the destination—all efforts to seek emotional balance will have tremendous health benefits.

Your path to being well depends on a take-charge attitude and health-supportive changes according to *your* individual needs. Ultimately, I know that a holistic approach will help you *be well.* The next step is yours.

Chapter Notes

1. "2013 Report on the Health of Canadians," *Heart and Stroke Foundation, Heartandstroke.com,* accessed September 20, 2014, http://www.heartandstroke.com/atf/cf/%7B99452D8B-E7F1-4BD6-A57D-B136CE6C95BF%7D/Report-on-Cnd-Health--D17.pdf?_ga=1.133950286.1965050788.1346281094, 2.

APPENDIX 1: Bioenergetic Evaluation (BEE

Premises

Bioelectric energy, essential for human life, flows through meridians, a network of energetic pathways that pass through organs and tissues of the body. In Chinese medicine, this energy is called Qi (pronounced "chee").

The Bioenergetic Evaluation (BEE) tests the body's functional health through energy meridians. Testing also reveals how to restore balance to health.

Benefits

The BEE will reveal the status of your functional health. It will tell which meridians in your body are in balance, stressed, or weakened.

The BEE is a highly reliable test for food intolerances and sensitivities to additives and chemicals. The testing device sends out an electromagnetic signal to your body, which represents different foods, additives, or chemicals. Your body's response to these signals is measured. Studies have shown this testing as reliable as other methods (scratch allergy tests and blood tests).

The BEE can identify substances (foods, nutrition) that will support your body in functioning at a healthier level. When your body functions at a healthier level, you will be better able to cope with the challenge of disease.

How the BEE works

Readings are taken at specific "acu points" on the hands and feet to determine the functional status of each meridian. The readings will show whether the meridian and its associated organ and tissues are balanced, stressed, or weakened.

A brass rod is held in one hand while the technician uses a probe to take readings at prescribed points on your hands and feet. There is the possibility of mild discomfort from the probe pressed on the skin.

How BEE differs from medical treatment

The primary purpose of this system is to evaluate the energy flow through the body. It is not meant to make a medical diagnosis or replace medical intervention. BEE testing and balancing does not take the place of qualified medical diagnosis and treatment.

BEE testing is a way to address concerns that do not show up in other tests. It is helpful for those who want to improve their general health, as well as for those with chronic problems that lack a specific diagnosis or that have not responded to other treatment.

No Risk Test

The FDA (.U.S.) classifies this equipment as a "non-significant risk" device. The amount of electrical current used in BEE testing is in the range of millionths of an amp. This is so slight that you will not even feel it. Because this is a topical evaluation, it is noninvasive and completely safe.

This technology can be compared to a polygraph, EKG (electrocardiogram), EEG (electroencephalogram), EMG (electromyogram), MRI (magnetic resonance imaging), and other technologies that measure electrical response on the surface of the skin.

APPENDIX 2: Digestive Balancing Diet

Restores healthy digestive function, aids in weight loss and if food sensitivities are suspected. This diet can be followed for extended periods of time. Number of servings varies according to height and activity level.

Foods to Have:

Vegetables (3-4 /day): Organic; mix of dark green and orange; steamed or raw; fermented beets or pickles

Animal protein (1-3/day): Cold-water fish, free-range chicken and turkey, free-range eggs

Fruits (2/day): Organic; locally grown in season or frozen in winter

Grains (2-4/day): Rice (brown and basmati), quinoa, teff. If tolerated, oats, kamut, spelt, rye. Sourdough bread

Nuts (15-20 nuts/day) Raw almonds, walnuts, pine, pecans, and hazelnuts

Seeds(< ¼ cup/day): Raw sunflower, pumpkin and sesame seeds; tahini

Legumes (1/day): Adzuki, lentils, navy, hummus, black or split peas

Dairy (1-2 cups/day): Rice milk, almond milk, goat cheese. If dairy tolerant, organic plain yogurt and kefir

Oils (2-3 tbsp): Extra-virgin olive oil, flax oil (unheated); organic coconut oil; expeller-pressed oils; homemade salad dressing using extra-virgin olive oil, lemon, and seasonings

Sweeteners (1-3 tsp): Stevia, unpasteurized local honey, rice syrup

Other flavourings: Sea salt, most herbs and spices

Fluids (quantity per size & activity): Spring or filtered water, green tea, herbal teas

Foods to Avoid: More difficult to digest, destabilizing to gut flora; apt to contain additives that have negative health effects

Vegetables: Limit starchy vegetables such as potatoes. Nightshades: tomatoes, peppers, and eggplant

Animal protein: Beef, pork, cold cuts, bacon, sausage

Fruits: Fruits that tend to mold: strawberries, grapes, melons

Grains: Wheat, corn, yeasted breads, muffins, cookies, cakes, pies

Nuts: Peanuts, cashews, pistachios; all roasted nuts

Seeds: Roasted seeds

Legumes: Peanuts, peanut butter, lima beans, soybeans, and soy protein isolate

Dairy: Cow's milk, cheese from cow's milk, cream, ice cream

Oils: Butter, margarine, most cooking oils and salad dressings

Sweeteners: White sugar, corn syrup, high-fructose corn syrup, maple syrup

Other flavourings: Table salt

Fluids: Fruit juice, coffee, soft drinks, alcohol

Other: Fried and deep-fried foods; MSG; aspartame; nitrates, sulphites, food dyes; processed/packaged foods

APPENDIX 3: Alkaline Balancing Diet

Follow this diet after an illness or if the body is in an acidic state

Foods to comprise 70 percent of daily diet

Vegetables: All, except potatoes and mushrooms

Legumes: Lentils, lima beans, white navy beans

Fruits: Avocados; cherries, sour; coconut, fresh, unsweetened; grapefruit, lemons, limes, tomatoes

Grains: Buckwheat, millet, quinoa

Nuts: Almonds

Seeds: Caraway, cumin, fennel, pumpkin, sesame, sprouted seeds (alfalfa, red clover, and broccoli)

Oils: Avocado, borage, coconut, cod liver, evening primrose, flaxseed, marine lipids (fish oil), olive

Beverages: Alkaline water, water with fresh lemon, fresh vegetable juice, almond milk, unsweetened

Herbs and Spices: Celtic sea salt, Himalayan salt, cayenne pepper, red pepper flakes, and most other herbs and spices, except curry, nutmeg, vanilla

Foods to comprise no more than 30 per cent of daily diet

Proteins: Organic – beef, poultry, eggs, organ meats; freshwater fish (wild); wild caught ocean fish

Fruits: Apples, apricots, bananas, berries, cantaloupe, cherries (sweet), currents, dates (fresh), figs (fresh), grapes, Honeydew melon, mangos, nectarines, oranges, papaya, peaches, pineapple, tangerines, watermelon, and dried fruit preserved with sulfites

Grains: Amaranth, barley, brown rice, kamut, kasha, millet, oatmeal, oat bran, rye, triticale, wild rice

Legumes: Black beans, chickpeas, kidney beans

Nuts (fresh, raw, and refrigerated): Brazil, cashews, hazelnuts, peanuts, pecans, pistachios, walnuts

Seeds: (fresh, raw, and refrigerated): flaxseeds, sunflower

Dairy: Rice milk, unsweetened (without casein, sweeteners, preservatives, hydrogenated fats, or trans fats)

Oils: Canola, organic, cold pressed; grape seed; sunflower

Sweeteners: Barley malt syrup, brown rice syrup, cane juice, unpasteurized honey, maple syrup, organic, unrefined sugar cane

Beverages: Black or green tea; coffee (not decaffeinated), fruit juice (unsweetened, no preservatives, additives or colours)

Herbs and Spices: Organic, unsweetened cocoa and carob; curry, nutmeg, vanilla

Foods to eat rarely

Vegetables: Mushrooms, potatoes

Proteins: Non-organic beef, veal, pork, organ meats, poultry, eggs; shellfish, farmed fish

Fruits: Canned fruit of all kinds, pickled fruit, fruit syrups, jam, jelly, pie filling

Grains: White flour, baked goods containing white flour, white bread, multigrain bread made with white flour, rye bread made with white flour, whole-wheat bread or pasta, whole-grain bread, white rice

Dairy: Cow's milk, cream, hard cheese, cottage cheese, ice cream, yogurt, soy cheese, goat's milk/cheese, whey, casein

Oils: Margarine, butter, clarified butter, corn oil

Nuts and seeds: Roasted nuts, salted nuts, all unrefrigerated nuts, most packaged nuts

Sweeteners: White sugar, refined sugar, brown sugar, turbinado sugar, fructose, corn syrup, pasteurized honey

Beverages: Alcohol, beer, wine, fruit juice, sweetened

Extras: Ketchup, malt, mayonnaise, monosodium glutamate, mustard, vinegar, soy sauce, table salt, yeast

Sources: Gates, Colbin, Schoffro Cook, http://www.alkaline-alkaline.com/ph_food_chart.html

APPENDIX 4: Anti-Inflammatory Diet

Eat larger meals at breakfast and lunch. No food within three hours of bedtime. Some foods have direction on the minimum and maximum number of servings per week. Daily servings depend on body size and activity level. See the Digestive Balancing Diet in Appendix 1 for serving ranges.

Foods to Have:

Steamed, Juiced Vegetables—mix of dark green and orange daily.

Organic, locally grown is ideal. *If not juicing*, limit raw vegetables to soft ones such as lettuce and avocado.

Animal Proteins—Eaten at breakfast and lunch *only*.

Eggs, free range, 3-5 servings per week: Soft-boiled or raw, i.e., pour hot tap water over the egg and leave for 5 minutes

Fish, 4 servings per week: Deep-sea fish (wild Pacific salmon, halibut, cod, sardines, trout, and mackerel)

Chicken/Turkey: Organic or free range; white meat only. Do not eat the skin.

Undenatured whey protein OR vegan protein powder – one serving daily

Fruit—Eat *before* or *between* meals

Whole fruit, organic: Apple, berries, cranberry, lemon, lime, peaches, pears, plums, watermelon.

No raw fruit in presence of diarrhea.

Whole Grains: Brown rice, quinoa, millet

Legumes: Fermented soy (tempeh, miso), northern, white, green, string; sprouted mung bean

Nuts: Raw, unsalted: Soak overnight before eating, almonds, Brazil nuts, walnuts, cashews

Seeds: Raw, unsalted sunflower, pumpkin, sesame; sprouted alfalfa

Fats/Oils: Flax, ground; extra-virgin olive oil (e.g., homemade salad dressing). Expeller-pressed oils; "Better butter"—mix flax oil with ghee (clarified butter)

Dairy or alternatives: Rice or almond milk; goat cheese; organic yogurt or kefir, if dairy tolerant

Sweeteners: Stevia, natural unpasteurized honey, rice syrup

Other flavorings: Sea salt in small quantities

Fluids: Spring or filtered water. Squeeze half lemon into one glass before breakfast. Herbal teas: Dandelion, sage, milk thistle, cinnamon or chicory herb tea; green tea

Other: Apple cider vinegar (Bragg brand; substitute for Worcestershire sauce), plain mustard

Avoid the following:

Cow's milk, cheese, cream, ice cream, yogurt with fruit or sugar

Red meat, pork, deli meats, smoked meats, sausages, bacon, shellfish

Grains (cereals, bread, crackers, cakes, cookies, flour): wheat, corn, oats, rye, kamut, spelt, barley, buckwheat

Citrus fruits and fruit that tends to mold, i.e., grapes, melons, strawberries

Peanuts and peanut butter, pistachios, cashews

All caffeinated foods: teas, coffee, chocolate

Fruit juices

Sugar, alcohol, artificial sweeteners (aspartame, sorbitol, sucralose)

White vinegar

Table salt; cayenne pepper; others as tolerated

Fried foods of any kind; margarine; mayonnaise (unless made with expeller-pressed oils)

Additives: MSG, BHT, nitrates, nitrites, sulfites, food dyes

Restaurant food: Tends to have additives and damaged fats

APPENDIX 5: Glycemic Values of Carbohydrates

Carbohydrate foods with a low-glycemic index will break down slowly so that blood sugar is not greatly affected. This prevents hunger and cravings, which leads to overeating. Low-glycemic index (GI) foods are recommended for weight control and for those with blood sugar regulation issues (hypoglycemics, diabetics).

This list includes fruits, grains, legumes, and a few vegetables. *All other vegetables* have a low GI, and are therefore okay. (Source: Brand-Miller et al)

Low GI (<55): BEST FOODS

Lentils, green, canned 52
Porridge, oatmeal 49
Orange 43
Black-eyed beans 41
Apple juice 41
Corn hominy (Grits) 40
Pinto beans 39
Apple 36
Yogurt, low fat, fruit 33
Chick peas (garbanzo beans) 33
Split peas, yellow, boiled 32
Lima beans, baby, frozen 32
Black beans 30

Kidney beans, dried 29
Lentils, green 29
Peach 28
Lentils 28
Lentils, red 25
Barley, pearled 25
Grapefruit 25
Peas, dried 22
Rice Bran 19
Soya beans 18
Peanuts 15

Moderate GI (56-69): FOODS IN MODERATION

Barley bread 65
Rye bread 65
Macaroni and Cheese 64
Beets 64
Raisins 64
Black bean soup 64
Pizza, cheese 60
Split pea soup 60
Spaghetti, white 59
Papaya 58
Mango 56
Buckwheat 55

Sweet corn 55
Rice (high amylose, Basmati) 50-60
Sweet potato 55
Kidney beans, canned 55
Banana 53
Pineapple 52
Orange juice 52
Peas, green 50
Baked beans (canned) 50
Carrots 50

High GI (>70) GI rating: FOODS TO AVOID

Potatoes 100
Soft drink, Fanta, Coke, etc. 97
Bread, white, French 95
Rice, white 90
French bread 95
Ice cream 87
Breakfast cereals, Cornflakes, 85
Pretzels 81
Jelly beans, candy 80
Whole-wheat bread 75
French fries 75
Pumpkin 75
Graham Wafers 74
Millet 71
Rice, brown (instant) 70
Cream of Wheat 70
Cornmeal, cornbread 69

BIBLIOGRAPHY

A Course in Miracles, Combined Volume, Workbook, Third edition. Mill Valley, California: Foundation for Inner Peace, 2007.

Agus, Dr. David B. *The End of Illness.* New York, New York: Free Press, 2011.

Armstrong, Karen. *12 Steps to a Compassionate Life.* New York, New York: Anchor Books, 2010.

Atkins, Robert C., MD. *Dr. Atkins' New Diet Revolution: The Amazing No-Hunger Weight-Loss Plan That Has Helped Millions Lose Weight and Keep It Off.* New York, New York: Avon Books, 1992.

Atkinson, William W. *Thought Vibration, or the Law of Attraction in the Thought World.* New York, New York: Cosimo Books, 2006, originally published in 1906.

Balch, James and Phyllis Balch. *Prescription for Nutritional Healing,* Second edition. Garden City Park, New York: Avery Publishing, 1997.

Ballantyne, Rudolph, MD. *Diet & Nutrition: A Holistic Approach.* Honesdale, Pennsylvania: The Himalayan International Institute, 1978.

Barnard, Neal D., MD and Bryanna Grogan. *Dr. Neal Barnard's Program for Reversing Diabetes: The Scientifically Proven System for Reversing Diabetes without Drugs.* New York, New York: Rodale Books, 2007.

Bateson-Koch, Carolee, DC, ND. *Allergies: Disease in Disguise.* Burnaby, British Columbia: Alive Books, 1994.

Beliveau, Richard, PhD and Denis Gringras, PhD. *Foods That Fight Cancer: Preventing Cancer through Diet.* Toronto, Ontario: McClelland & Stewart, 2005.

Bergner, Paul. *The Healing Power of Minerals, Special Nutrients and Trace Elements.* San Diego, California: Prima Publishing, 1977.

Blaylock, Russell, L., MD. *Excitotoxins: The Taste That Kills.* Albuquerque, New Mexico: Health Press NA, 1997.

Bowen, Will. *A Complaint Free World: How to Stop Complaining and Start Enjoying the Life You Always Wanted.* New York, New York: Doubleday, 2007.

Brand-Miller, Jennie et al. *The Glucose Revolution: The Authoritative Guide to the Glycemic Index—The Groundbreaking Medical Discovery.* New York, New York: Marlowe and Company, 1996.

Budwig, Dr. Johanna. *Flax Oil as a True Aid against Arthritis, Heart Infarction, Cancer and Other Diseases.* Vancouver, British Columbia: Apple Publishing Co., 1992.

Campbell, T. Colin, PhD and Thomas M. Campbell II. *The China Study: Startling Implications for Diet, Weight Loss and Long-Term Health.* Dallas, Texas: Benbella Books, 2006.

Chopra, Deepak, MD. *Grow Younger, Live Longer.* New York, New York: Harmony Books, 2001.

___. *Reinventing the Body, Resurrecting the Soul: How to Create a New You.* New York, New York: Harmony Books, 2009.

Colbin, Annemarie. *Food and Healing,* Tenth anniversary edition. New York, New York: Ballantyne Books, 1996.

D'Adamo, Dr. Peter J. *Change your Genetic Destiny.* New York, New York: Broadway Books, 2007.

___. *Eat Right 4 Your Type.* New York, New York: Berkeley Publishing Group, 2002.

David, Marc. *The Slow Down Diet: Eating for Pleasure, Energy and Weight Loss.* Rochester, Vermont: Healing Arts Press, 2005.

Davis, William, MD. *Wheat Belly: Lose the Wheat, Lose the Weight, and Find Your Way Back to Health.* New York, New York: Rodale Books, 2011.

Dyer, Wayne W. *The Power of Intention: Learning to Co-create Your World Your Way.* Carlsbad, California: Hay House, 2004.

___. *There's a Spiritual Solution to Every Problem.* California: HarperCollins Publishers, 2003.

Erasmus, Udo. *Fats That Heal, Fats That Kill.* Burnaby, British Columbia: Alive Books, 1993.

Fallon, Sally with Mary G. Enig, PhD. *Nourishing Traditions,* Revised 2nd edition. Washington, DC: New Trends Publishing Inc., 2001.

Francis, Raymond, MSc. *Never Be Sick Again: Health Is a Choice, Learn How to Choose It.* Deerfield Beach, Florida: Health Communications, Inc., 2002.

Fuhrman, Joel, MD. *Eat to Live: The Amazing Nutrient-Rich Program for Fast and Sustained Weight Loss,* Second edition. New York, New York: Little, Brown and Company, 2013.

Gates, Donna. *Body Ecology Diet: Recovering Your Health and Rebuilding Your Immunity.* Carlsbad, California: Hay House Inc., 2010.

Gittleman, Ann Louise, MS, CNS. *How to Stay Young and Healthy in a Toxic World.* Los Angeles, California: Keats Publishing, 1999.

Hawkins, David, MD, PhD. *Power vs. Force: The Hidden Determinants of Human Behavior.* Carlsbad, California: Hay House Inc., 1995.

Hay, Louise. *You Can Heal Your Life*. Carlsbad, California: Hay House, 1999.

Hill, Napoleon. *Think and Grow Rich*. New York, New York: Ballantine Publishing, 1960.

Hoffer, Dr. Abram, MD, FRCP with Linus Pauling, PhD. *Healing Cancer: Complementary Vitamin and Drug Treatments*. Toronto, Ontario: Canadian College of Naturopathic Medicine Press, 2004.

Jensen, Dr. Bernard and Mark Anderson. *Empty Harvest: Understanding the Link between Our Food, Our Immunity and Our Planet*. New York, New York: Penguin Putnam Inc., 1990.

Junger, Alejandro, MD. *Clean Gut: The Breakthrough Plan for Eliminating the Root Cause of Disease and Revolutionizing Your Health*. New York, New York: Harper Collins Publishers, 2013.

Laidlaw, Stuart. *Secret Ingredients: The Brave New World of Industrial Farming*. Toronto, Ontario: McClelland & Stewart, 2003.

Lipton, Bruce H., PhD. *The Biology of Belief: Unleashing the Power of Consciousness, Matter & Miracles*. Santa Rosa, California: Mountain of Love/Elite Books, 2005.

Lustig, Robert H., MD. *Fat Chance: Beating the Odds Against Sugar, Processed Foods, Obesity and Disease*. New York, New York: Hudson Street Press, Penguin Group, 2013.

MacWilliams, Lyle, Bsc, Msc, FP. *Comparative Guide to Nutritional Supplements,* 3rd edition. Vernon, British Columbia: Northern Dimensions Publishing, 2003.

Martin, Jeanne Marie with Rona, Zoltan P., MD. *Complete Candida Yeast Guidebook: Everything You Need to Know about Prevention, Treatment & Diet,* Revised 2nd edition. Roseville, California: Prima Publishing, 2000.

Matsen, John, ND. *Eating Alive: Prevention Thru Good Digestion*. North Vancouver, British Columbia: Compton Books, 2002.

Matthews-Simonton, Stephanie with Robert L. Shook. *The Healing Family: The Simonton Approach for Families Facing Illness*. New York, New York: Bantam Books, 1984.

McManners, Dr. Deborah. *The Ultimate Holistic Health Book: Your Guide to Ultimate Health & Well-Being,* 2nd edition. London, England: Piatkus Books, 2006.

McTaggart, Lynne. *The Intention Experiment: Using Your Thoughts to Change Your Life and the World*. New York, New York: Free Press, 2007.

Moore Lappe, Frances. *Diet for a Small Planet*. New York, New York: Ballantine Books, 1971.

Murray, Michael, ND, Joseph Pizzorno, ND and Lara Pizzorno, MA, LMT. *The Encyclopedia of Healing Foods*. New York: New York: Pocket Books, 2005.

Myss, Carolyn, PhD. *Anatomy of the Spirit: The Seven Stages of Power and Healing*. New York, New York: Three Rivers Press, 1996.

___. *Why People Don't Heal and How They Can*. New York, New York: Three Rivers Press, 1997.

Nestle, Marion. *Food Politics: How the Food Industry Influences Nutrition and Health*. Oakland, California: University of California Press, 2007.

Ornish, Dr. Dean, MD. *Dr. Dean Ornish's Program for Reversing Heart Disease: The Only System Scientifically Proven to Reverse Heart Disease without Drugs or Surgery*. New York, New York: Ballantyne Books, 1990.

Peale, Norman Vincent. *The Power of Positive Thinking*. New York, New York: Prentice-Hall, Inc., 1952.

Pelton, Ross, RPh and James B. LaValle, RPh. *The Nutritional Cost of Prescription Drugs: How to Maintain Good Nutrition While Using Prescription Drugs*. Englewood, Colorado: Morton Publishing Company, 2000.

Perrault, Danielle, RHN. *Nutritional Symptomatology*. Richmond Hill, Ontario: CSNN Publishing, a division of the Canadian School of Natural Nutrition, 2000.

Pollan, Michael. *Food Rules: An Eater's Manual*. New York, New York: Penguin Press, 2009.

___. *In Defense of Food: An Eater's Manifesto*. New York, New York: Penguin Press, 2008.

Pritikin, Nathan. *The Pritikin Permanent Weight-Loss Manual*. New York, New York: Bantam Books, 1981.

Roberts, Wayne, Rod MacRae and Lori Stahlbrand. *Real Food for a Change: Bringing Nature, Joy and Justice to the Table*. Toronto, Ontario: Random House, 1999.

Rona, Zoltan P., MD. *Natural Alternatives to Vaccination*. Vancouver, British Columbia: Alive Books, 2000.

Schmidt, Dr. Michael A., Dr. Lendon H. Sennet and Dr. Keith W. Sennet. *Beyond Antibiotics: 50 (or so) Ways to Boost Immunity and Avoid Antibiotics*. Berkeley, California: North Atlantic Books, 1993.

Schoffro Cook, Michelle, DNM, DAc, CNC. *The Ultimate pH Solution: Balance Your Body Chemistry to Prevent Disease and Lose Weight*. Toronto, Ontario: Harper Collins, 2008.

Schroeder, Henry A., MD. *The Poisons Around Us: The Unseen Dangers in Our Air, Water, Cookware and Food, and Their Leading Roles in Sickness and Death.* Chicago, Illinois: Keats Publishing, 1978.

Schwarcz, Joe, PhD. *An Apple A Day: The Myths, Misconceptions, and Truths About the Foods We Eat.* Toronto, Ontario: HarperCollins, 2007.

Siegel, Bernie S., MD. *The Art of Healing: Uncovering Your Inner Wisdom and Potential for Self-Healing.* Novato, California: New World Library, 2013

____. *Love, Medicine and Miracles: Lessons Learned about Self-Healing from a Surgeon's Experience with Exceptional Patients.* New York, New York: Harper & Row, 1986.

Stadler Mitrea, Lilieana, MD(Eur), ND, DNM. *Pathology and Nutrition: A Guide for Professionals,* First edition revised. Richmond Hill, Ontario: CSNN Publishing, a division of the Canadian School of Natural Nutrition, 2005.

Suneja, Ashima, ND. *Essentials of Nutritional Immunology.* Uxbridge, Ontario: CSNN Publishing, 2007

Tolle, Eckhart. *A New Earth: Awakening to Your Life's Purpose.* New York, New York: Penguin Books, 2006.

Trivieri, Larry and The American Holistic Medical Association. *Guide to Holistic Health: Healing Therapies for Optimal Wellness.* New York, New York: John Wiley & Sons, 2001.

Vanderhaeghe, Lorna and Patrick Bouic, PhD. *The Immune System Cure: Nature's Way to Super-Powered Health.* Toronto, Ontario: Prentice Hall Canada, 1999.

Walker, Dr. Ross. *Highway to Health: Antioxidants and You.* Cape Town, Republic of South Africa: Dream House Publishing, 2000.

Williams, Roger J., PhD. *Biochemical Individuality: The Basis of the Genotrophic Concept.* New Canaan, Connecticut: Keats Publishing, 1998.

Williamson, Marianne. *A Course in Weight Loss: 21 Spiritual Lessons for Surrendering Your Weight Forever.* Carlsbad, California: Hay House, 2010.

____. *The Gift of Change: Spiritual Guidance for a Radically New Life.* San Francisco, California: Harper Books, 2004.

Wollcott, William L. and Trish Fahey. *The Metabolic Typing Diet: Customize Your Diet for: Permanent Weight Loss, Optimal Health, Preventing and Reversing Disease, Staying Young at Any Age.* New York, New York: Broadway Books, 2000.

INDEX

185; emotional stress, 68,117;
infections, 56, 59, 113, 140, 165,
167,170, irritable bowel syndrome,
122-3; medication effects, 118, 122;
nutrient deficits, 6, 21; 153;
sensitivities, 36, 37, 93-4, 95, 97;
supplements, 152; toxicity, 176, 177
Digestive processes, 24, 68, 82, 87, 112,
116, 162, 178
support for, 58, 73, 82, 83, 88, 114,
130, 140, 141, 143, 152, 154, 169
Dysbiosis, 124, 163-4, 166, 167
healing for, 169-170

E

Echinacea, 152, 168
Eczema, 37, 127, 131, 164, 174
Edema, 37, 93
-   see also Water retention
Eggs, 74, 130, 140
and cholesterol, 41-2; blood type
diet, 91; in healing diet, 167; in
quality diet, 74; sensitivity, 94; in
vegetarian diet, 88
Electroencephalogram (EEG), 6, 121
Electrocardiogram (EKG), 6, 121
Elimination processes, 5, 79, 112, 116,
129, 162
diet 92, 94, 95, 97; exercise, 83, 114;
healing, 115, 137, 139, 140, 154, 168-
170, 175-8; medication effects, 118;
malfunction, 97, 115, 128, 129, 163,
172, 173, 174; pathways in the body,
124, 173, 176, 177
Elimination protocol, 95-6
Emotional Freedom Technique, 108
Environmental Protection Agency (EPA), 12,
15, 51, 54, 55
Enzymes, digestive, 125, 126, 128, 162
supplements, 115, 145, 152, 170;
depletion, 15, 53, 118, 135, 153
Enzymes in food, 17, 36, 137, 140
E. coli (*Escherichia coli*), 36, 59, 163
Epigenetics, 7, 85, 91, 92, 179
Essential fatty acids, 21, 32, 40, 76, 115,
116, 155, 158
Estrogen, 36, 43, 44
Exercise, 83-4, 91, 113, 129, 130, 181
in elimination protocol, 175; in
healing, 114-5, 120, 136, 142, 170

F

Fat, body, 76, 87, 89, 90, 175
in blood, 22, 41; in cells, 52, 177; in
tissue, 25, 178
Fats, dietary, 30, 76-7, 82, 86, 87, **89-90**,
93, 138, 143, 175
cooking with, 17, 80-81; in cow's
milk, 36; damaged, 2, 41, 45, 75, 77,
81, 124; health effects, 32, 36, 40-41,
76, 88, 90, 130, 131, 138, 154;
healthy sources, 75, 76-77, 88, 130;
heart disease, 33, 38-41, 76, 90;
homogenized, 36; hydrogenated, 38;
omega-3's and 6's, 76, 77;
polyunsaturated, 153; in processed
food, 20, 25, 26, 32, 136, 146;
saturated, 35, 38-41, 90; trans fats,
39-41, 45, 75, 77, 84, 112, 124
Fat metabolism, 5, 87, 100, 127, 135,
143, 158
Fatigue, 6, **129-30**
acidity, 135; infections, 58, 122, 130,
165; dietary influences, 21, 81, 91,
93, 100, 142; headaches, 130;
intestinal imbalance, 128; nutrient
deficit, 88; healing protocols, 138,
139, 167, 170; toxicity, 174, 175, 176,
177
-   see also Chronic Fatigue
Syndrome
Fertility, 176
Fever, 58, 59, 118, 119, 131
Fibre, 21, 40, 75, 120, 126, 140, 141, 175
Fibromyalgia, 24, 164
Fish, 74-5, 86
healing diet, 167; nutrients, 38, 88,
130, 135, 153; shellfish allergy, 94;
toxins, 26, 51, 53, 75
Flame retardants, 49, 52-3
Flax, 76, 88, 120, 135, 167, 175
Fluids, 78-9, 82
toxins, 16; role in healing, 120, 126,
129, 134
Fluoride, 53-4, 78, 83
Food and Drug Administration, 16, 17, 26
Formaldehyde, 24, 52, 57
Free radicals, 115, 142, 151, 152, 153
Fructose, 73
-   see also High-fructose corn syrup
Fruits, 73-4, 75, 86, 87, 91
additives, 23, 25, 26; 44, 45; in
healing diets, 120, 135, 136, 137, 138,
139, 140, 168, 175; juice from, 139,
168; nutrient content, 4, 11, 15, 16,

Indigestion – see Digestive malfunction.
Inflammation, 44, 124, 136-7, 143, 153, 166
Inositol – See Vitamins, individual
Insomnia
    chronic fatigue syndrome, 123; diet, 21, 93; emotional stress, 69, 117; parasites, 165; support for, 143
Intestinal imbalance, 125, **128-9**, 132, 134, 175
-    see also Dysbiosis
Intolerance – see Sensitivity
Irritable bowel disease, 61, 69, 140, 162, 165
Irritable bowel syndrome, 4, 17, 61, 69, 86, 122, 123, 134, 140, 165
Irritability, 59, 92, 119, 125, 165, 176
Isopropyl Alcohol, 54

J-K-L

Journaling, 95, 96, 108, 129
Kamut, 75, 89
Kidney disease, 22, 42, 51, 118
Kidney functions, 162, 173, 177
Kidney stones, 43, 142, 155
Kidney stress, 125, **127-8**
    acidity, 136; diet ,79, 89; natural healing, 134, 177; toxins, 15, 50, 52, 59
Lactose, 35, 36, 92, 94
Lead, 49, 50-51, 54, 153, 172
Lecithin, 42
Legumes, **75-6**
    nutrients, 38, 130, 140, 151; alkalinity 136
Listeria, 36
Liver functions, 41, 162, 173, 177, 178
Liver stress, 125, **127**, 158, 162, 178
    acidity, 136; additives, 25; chronic fatigue syndrome, 124; diet effects, 21, 79, 89, 142; disease, 23; healing support, 134, 151, 168, 169, 175, 176, 177; Irritable bowel syndrome, 123; malabsorption, 129, 158; medications, 132; parasites, 166; toxins, 51, 52, 55, 152
Lymph congestion – see Congestion
Lymph system, 173, 174

M

Magnesium, 12, 38, 42, 78, 118, 148, 155, 158, 168

Magnetic resonance imaging, 6, 121
Malabsorption, 5, 60, 69, 94, 96, 113, 115, 116, 117, 118, 124, 129, 130, 135, 137, 151, 158, 159, 163
Manganese, 38, 148, 155, 156
Margarine – see Fats, dietary
Meat, 31, 39, 74-5, 153
    acidity, 136, 142; contaminants, 11, 26, 53, 80, 163; in healing diets, 135, 140; in weight loss, 89
Medications, 1, **117-9**, 134, 180
    acid reflux, 122-123; anti-inflammatory, 123, 162; cholesterol lowering, 42, 132; natural healing, 112, 113, 18, 119, 120, 170; interactions, 136, 152; nutrient depletion, 154; pain, 124; preservatives, 26; side effects, 117, 118-119, 122, 123, 127, 128, 131, 132, 136, 163; toxins, 50
Meditation, 108, 109, 123
Memory, 76, 103
Memory loss, 21, 50, 52, 59, 88, 123, 165, 176
Meningitis, 57, 59, 121
Mercury
    sources, 51, 57, 74, 175; health effects, 49, 50, 51, 172; nutrient depletion, 153
Metabolic function, 114, 115, 130, 141, 151, 152, 158, 172
Metabolic typing diets, 91-2
Metabolism, 5, 112, 127
    dietary support, 76, 81-2, 136, faulty, 5, 87, 126, 130, 135; medications 118; overweight 87; supplements
Micronutrients, 115, 116, 145, 146, 148, 149, 151, 153, 156
Migraines – see Headaches
Milk, cow's, **35-38**
    additives, 23, and bone health, 38; as calcium source, 37-38; fermentation, 141; in infant formula, 36; in quality diet, 77-8; raw, 140; sensitivity, 37, 44, 86, 87, 92, 94, 96; in vegetarian diet, 88
Milk thistle, 175
Minerals
    absorption, 5, 38, 42-3, 151, 157, 158; bone health 38, 156, 157; deficiencies 69, 146, 154, 155; dietary sources 11, 17, 22, 38, 73, 75, 79, 80, 129, 136, 140; fluids78-79; health

www.ingramcontent.com/pod-product-compliance
Lightning Source LLC
Chambersburg PA
CBHW072131270326
41931CB00010B/1731